'Metabolism, inflammation, and immunity are three sides of the same coin. Fix one and you fix them all. Dr Aseem Malhotra offers you a way to fix all three at once, and the solution is as easy as your fork.'

Dr Robert Lustig, *New York Times* bestselling author of *Fat Chance*

'A crystal-clear roadmap to reverse the root causes of our poor metabolic and immune health. It is the handbook of health for our time.'

Dr Mark Hyman, *New York Times* bestselling author of *Food Fix*

'I've been unfortunate enough to have had #COVID19. I feel had I not focused on regaining my metabolic health and sending my type 2 diabetes into remission things could have been much worse. This amazing doctor puts his head above the parapet. I have great respect for Dr Aseem Malhotra and owe my regained metabolic health to him.'

Debra Scott, retired civil servant

'Feel good today and increase your chance of living a longer and healthier life. In this well researched book Dr Malhotra provides the science and the steps for this double win.'

Dr Campbell Murdoch, Clinical Adviser, Royal College of General Practitioners

The 21-Day Immunity Plan

How to Rapidly Improve Your Metabolic Health and Resilience to Fight Infection

Dr Aseem Malhotra

First published in Great Britain in 2020 by Yellow Kite
An imprint of Hodder & Stoughton
An Hachette UK company

14

Copyright © Aseem Malhotra 2020

The right of Aseem Malhotra to be identified as the Author of the Work has been
asserted by him in accordance with the Copyright, Designs and Patents Act 1988.

A CIP catalogue record for this title is available from the British Library

Paperback ISBN 978 1 529 34967 2
eBook ISBN 978 1 529 34968 9

Typeset in Celeste by Hewer Text UK Ltd, Edinburgh
Printed and bound in Great Britain by Clays Ltd, Elcograf S.p.A.

Hodder & Stoughton policy is to use papers that are natural, renewable
and recyclable products and made from wood grown in sustainable
forests. The logging and manufacturing processes are expected to
conform to the environmental regulations of the country of origin.

Yellow Kite
Hodder & Stoughton Ltd
Carmelite House
50 Victoria Embankment
London EC4Y 0DZ

www.yellowkitebooks.co.uk

I dedicate this book to my late mother Dr Anisha Malhotra and my father Dr Kailash Chand Malhotra for their love, unwavering support, kindness and through example teaching me the true meaning of compassion.

Disclaimer

This book is not a replacement for working with your healthcare professionals who know your specific circumstances. All matters, treatments and specific questions regarding your health care should be discussed with your GP or a suitably qualified medical person. The author and publisher disclaim any liability directly or indirectly from the use of the material in this book by any person.

Contents

Foreword

Dr Aseem Malhotra is a quite remarkable man. He's a consultant cardiologist who took a step back and asked himself why more and more people were getting cardiovascular disease. As well as treating his patients' conditions, he took time to think very deeply about how he could prevent people from falling sick in the first place.

His first book, *The Pioppi Diet*, was a result of these reflections. It helped me on a health journey that led me to lose eight stone in weight, reduce my blood pressure and reverse type 2 diabetes.

His approach to helping people get well is to explain to them, without judgement, that the system is stacked against them; that the obesogenic environment makes it almost impossible to avoid sugary, ultra-processed food. Just think about this for a moment: we serve burgers, chips and ice-cream to heart patients in NHS hospitals. Our kids can buy donuts in school. You can buy a pumpkin spiced latte in a high-street coffee shop with more than 14 teaspoons of sugar in it. When you pause and think about it, you realise how crazy that is.

So it's not all your fault if you suffer from conditions related to excess body fat, best determined by your metabolic health, which affects even many of those with a so-called normal body weight. But to get well and stay well, there are lifestyle changes you have to make. And let me tell you: if you take Aseem's advice on how to balance your nutrition, become more active and manage your stress, you stand a good chance of living a longer, healthier and more fulfilling life.

Britain was suffering an obesity epidemic prior to COVID-19 hitting us. Nearly 10% of the NHS budget is spent on treating type 2 diabetes alone. Yet research by organisations like Virta Health suggest that with a change of nutrition from the standard Western diet that is high in ultra-processed food and sugar, nearly half of those with type 2 diabetes can reverse their condition or significantly reduce the amount of medication they have to take.

Whether you reverse type 2 diabetes or reduce your blood glucose levels isn't just an academic exercise. You're actually getting your life back. You don't nod off in the middle of the afternoon. You take fewer trips to the bathroom in the middle of the night. You have more energy. You just feel better. And there are millions of people that can have this joy returning to their lives.

In the era of COVID-19, you have an even stronger argument to get well and return to good metabolic health. If you have high blood pressure, are overweight, or have type 2 diabetes, you stand more of a chance of being adversely affected by the virus. Nearly 8% of critically ill patients with COVID-19 in intensive care units have been morbidly obese, compared with 2.9% of the general population. Those are probabilities you want to reduce if you can.

And so, Aseem's timely, evidence-based and brilliant new 21-day immunity plan is a perfect way to take the first step to transforming your life. I wish you well on your journey to better health.

Tom Watson
Chair of UK Music and Former Deputy Leader of the Labour Party

Introduction

'In the midst of every crisis lies great opportunity.'
—*Albert Einstein*

When the UK prime minister, Boris Johnson, was admitted to hospital unwell from symptoms of COVID-19 in early April 2020, the country feared the worst. I had observed that a number of his slim colleagues who had also contracted the virus remained relatively well, managing to cope by self-isolating at home. But rather than coincidence, through analysing the published research and with my own knowledge as a doctor practising in the NHS for almost two decades, it was clear to me that people who were overweight and suffering from conditions associated with (but not exclusive to) obesity, were at significantly increased risk of complications and death, not just from COVID-19 but from many infections.

In early March, data from Italy, a country that had experienced high death rates from COVID-19, revealed that 99% of those that had died had been suffering from at least one chronic condition. Research published in the *Lancet* demonstrated that 60% of those that died in Wuhan, China, where the virus is thought to have originated, suffered from high blood pressure or type 2 diabetes.

What was missing from the mainstream media discussion and public health messaging surrounding the virus, was that the underlying root cause of these conditions is related to lifestyle (fuelled by the environments in which we grow, live and work) and that dietary changes alone, as my own clinical experience with patients had also demonstrated, could rapidly and substantially improve many of these risk factors.

After my comments that the prime minister's more severe experience of the illness was likely linked to his weight were widely publicised, the secretary of state for health and social care asked me to provide him with more detailed evidence linking COVID-19 with obesity. But I informed him, and as you will come to learn in reading this book, this was far from being an issue about obesity alone. It's about all the preventable and modifiable lifestyle factors that lead to an immune system that is not as resilient as it could be.

But aside from my ability to analyse and provide a medical response to the crisis, absorbing the unnecessary suffering and deaths of thousands of people from this potentially deadly contagion was something that had a very personal resonance with me too, and gave me an even greater incentive to write this book: the premature deaths of two family members who suffered and died because of a compromised immune system.

The first was the death of my older brother, Amit, who died of a virus that affected his heart at the age of 13. Born with Down's syndrome, his compromised immune system was genetic and there was little that could have been done to prevent his death from crashing heart failure when he caught a tummy bug that most people would have been able to fight off. The second was my mother, who over the four-week period of her final admission to hospital endured indescribable pain from an infection that affected her spine. Her compromised immune system was almost entirely rooted in lifestyle choices. Because the NHS was already overstretched, a heart attack was missed, treatment was delayed and she gasped for breath as fluid engulfed her lungs. Eventually she slipped into a coma, as the infection spread through her body and she passed away aged only 68.

Beyond my observations as a medical scientist and my duties as a clinical doctor to share knowledge on the link between metabolic health and immunity, I write this book with the perspective and motivation of someone who has had to deal with all the emotion and sadness of seeing a close family member die well before their time and in the most horrible of circumstances. No one needs to suffer like she did and no family member should have to witness it.

What COVID-19 has also done is expose areas in our health systems and personal well-being that have long been neglected, and in themselves have made us more vulnerable to such a particularly pernicious virus. But in spite of the tragedy, the disturbing statistics and heart-breaking stories that have collectively gripped the world, we can draw from the lessons the virus has taught us and look to a brighter future.

Reading this book will help you understand how so many people have lost their lives from the virus, but more importantly it is a practical guide to help you, your friends and your family support your immunity and optimise your resilience to fighting infection. Through science and lessons from history, I hope that it will also empower you to challenge the marketing messages and health misinformation that can make us overweight and sick, and that it will offer populations around the world a way forward, to significantly reduce the threat from this, and any future pandemic, again.

CHAPTER 1

What We've Learned About COVID-19

As of July 2020, COVID-19 has spread around the world to 200 countries with more than 10 million confirmed cases and well over half a million confirmed deaths.

A 'coronavirus' is a family of viruses that usually cause disease in animals. The explanation most often given for the origin of COVID-19 (short for COronaVIrus Disease 2019) is a wild animal food market in Wuhan, China, in November 2019 and in this instance, it is thought to have come from bats. Over decades a handful of these viruses has been transmitted to humans, usually causing cold-like symptoms. In some ways COVID-19 resembles SARS (severe acute respiratory distress syndrome), which spread to many parts of the globe in 2002–2003, infecting around 8,000 and causing 800 deaths. Because those who became infected were very sick it was easy to identify, control and contain SARS and the virus subsequently died out. What makes COVID-19 unique and more difficult to control, is that for the majority who contract it – at least 80 per cent – the symptoms are mild. There are also many who remain asymptomatic and are thus able to carry the virus and unknowingly spread it, most easily from droplets that are expelled through talking, coughing or sneezing. Personal hygiene through regular hand washing is a crucial component in reducing the risk of getting infected after having contact with the virus either through touching someone who is infected (shaking hands, for example) or touching a surface that has been exposed to the virus from human transmission. The most common symptoms are sore throat, dry cough, headache and fever; others reported include fatigue, muscle aches, stomach upset and runny nose. Loss of smell may be the only symptom in approximately 3% of people infected. In the remaining 20 per cent of people who get more severe symptoms – predominantly through difficulty breathing – some end up needing hospital treatment where the most common complications are pneumonia and acute respiratory distress syndrome (or ARDS), which affects 15%. In these cases, severe inflammation results in the lungs losing complete ability to function without mechanical ventilation. Other complications include liver and heart injury, heart failure, blood clots and even stroke. For those unwell enough to need intensive care after being hospitalised the death rate is as high as 40%.

Who is most at risk and why are there differing death rates in different regions?

Within the mortality-rate figures, there is considerable variation according to age. This varies from a 3 in 10,000 risk of death for those aged between 5 and 17 to almost 1 in 3 for those over the age of 85. Among those hospitalised, 74–86% are aged at least 50 years old.

After age the baseline health or underlying conditions of the individual is what has the most significant impact on risk of death. For example, the risk of death is 12 times higher for those with underlying conditions (which we'll discuss later) than those without.

How is it spread?

Another major cited factor for variation in death rates in different countries has been the speed and ability of governments to implement physical distancing policies, which is the most effective way to limit social contact and reduce both symptomatic and asymptomatic spread.

Once infected the average time for someone to experience symptoms is five days, with the overwhelming majority demonstrating symptoms within two weeks. The median time from developing symptoms for those who need to go to hospital is seven days.

It is estimated that up to 62% of transmission of the virus occurs in the pre-symptomatic phase – in other words, before people start to feel unwell. Taking this into consideration it's easy to understand that without adequate control measures the virus is able to spread undetected quite rapidly.

The World Health Organization (WHO) declared COVID-19 to be a 'public health emergency' on 30th January 2020, acknowledging at that point that the virus had been spread, albeit in small detected numbers, across the globe. A number of countries started to implement measures to contain the spread, which initially involved quarantining travellers coming from areas of the world known to be infected. The primary strategy of the British government to protect the NHS from being overwhelmed was lockdown.

The mantra was 'Stay at home, protect the NHS, save lives.' But even though the NHS was just about able to cope, Britain ended up having one of the highest death tolls in Europe. There are many postulated factors behind this: the introduction of lockdown later rather than sooner; lack of provision for large-scale and appropriate testing to identify communities at risk; a shortage of personal protective equipment (PPE) for many frontline NHS staff exposed to a high viral load; and last, but by no means least, underlying poor metabolic health. In total over 500 health workers have tragically lost their lives in the UK, which include doctors, nurses and allied health professionals.

What does the future hold?

There are thousands of viruses that our bodies fight off every year, and even after we've got to grips with COVID-19 it's very possible that another pandemic may hit us not so far in the future. So, how do we go about arming ourselves with the tools and the resilience to tackle a virus of this kind in the future? And can we help support our immunity so that as individuals we are better equipped to fight off infection in general?

As we will soon discover, the factor putting many of those worse affected by COVID-19 most at risk of being unwell and dying is preventable and rapidly reversible: it is chronic metabolic diseases. Similarly, what drove our NHS to become overstretched long before COVID-19 hit our shores was the increasing burden of diet-related diseases.

The UK was terribly unprepared because for far too long we've neglected public health. The message that would save millions from unnecessary misery and which the government should have been encouraging for years is: 'Eat real food, protect the NHS, save lives.'

After all, the problem of diet-related disease is not a new concept. It was 2004 when the WHO declared obesity to be a global epidemic – yet not only have we failed to curb it, it's now far worse than it ever was. And as I will detail throughout the book, obesity itself is only the tip of the diet- and lifestyle-related disease iceberg.

The current primary focus for COVID-19 is to devise a vaccine as quickly as possible but based on what we know about influenza, a vaccine is likely to have some limitations in its effectiveness and impact if significant swathes of the population remain obese and or metabolically unhealthy.

But before we get into how we can rapidly reverse the risk factors for developing more severe illness and have better functioning global healthcare systems in the future, it's essential to understand and acknowledge what those barriers to progress have been.

How much do you know about the contribution of public health to our own sense of well-being and longevity? And how is this relevant to our immune system?

CHAPTER 2

Prevention is the Cure

'Prevention is not just better than cure, prevention IS the cure'

—*Professor Robert Lustig*

History has revealed that the largest determinant of health and longevity has very little to do with what happens within the walls of hospitals and a lot to do with what's going on outside in the community. In the UK, life expectancy has stopped increasing since 2010 and last year the British Heart Foundation revealed that for the first time in 50 years there has been an increase in death rates from cardiovascular disease in the under 75s.

The global health challenge of today is how to tackle the increasing burden of chronic disease that results in premature death and misery for tens of millions of people every year, not to mention the great stress it is placing on our healthcare systems.

Most of these chronic conditions, which include heart disease, type 2 diabetes, high blood pressure and even cancer and dementia, are rooted in poor metabolic health.

What is metabolic health?

In the simplest terms, metabolic health is best understood as the state of balance the body maintains between storing fat and burning it for energy. Once this balance is disrupted, health is adversely affected.

It is measured using five markers: blood glucose levels; blood pressure; waist circumference; and cholesterol profile, which is determined by the body's levels of triglycerides – a type of harmful fat found in the blood – and high-density lipoprotein (HDL-C), a beneficial cholesterol-carrying molecule.

Poor metabolic health is directly linked to the development of heart disease, type 2 diabetes and stroke, i.e., if the markers are at the wrong levels we are at greater risk of developing these diseases. Poor metabolic health is also linked to the development of cancer and dementia, and those with metabolic syndrome and its associated conditions are particularly vulnerable to complications from infections.

As we'll demonstrate in the next chapter, medical management can often be no better than putting a plaster on a severed artery, but there is a better way to rapidly reduce the risk of and in many cases bring our levels of these markers back to normal levels within a very short space of time. In fact, through very specific lifestyle changes, we can significantly improve and potentially normalise the levels within as little as 21 days.

This is not to undermine in any way the importance of surgery or medical treatment. If we treat 100,000 people for certain types of heart attack every year the procedure itself (known as emergency coronary stenting) will save or significantly extend the lives of 2,500, which is no small figure. But on an individual level,

Metabolic health markers – the measurements
An individual is considered to have optimal metabolic
health if their markers meet the following levels:
Average blood glucose (HbA1c) levels of less than 5.7%
Blood pressure lower than 120/80mmHg
Waist circumference of less than 102cm for a man; 88cm
for a woman (for South Asians it's less than 90cm for a
man; 85cm for a woman)
Blood triglycerides levels that are less than 1.7mmol/litre
(< 150md/dl)
High-density lipoprotein cholesterol (HDL-C) levels
that are greater than 1mmol/litre (> 40mg/dl in men
and > 50mg/dl in women)
A person is considered to have **metabolic syndrome**
when they fail to meet three of these optimal values,
meaning for example that someone who has high blood
pressure, high blood glucose and high triglycerides
would be considered to be at the highest risk of experi-
encing health problems.

carrying out emergency stenting during a heart attack only offers a
1 in 40 chance of the individual's life being saved. I always tell every
heart disease patient with a history of smoking that quitting their
habit will be more powerful in reducing the risk of a future heart
attack and death than all the medications they're taking combined.

Much, if not most, of medical care is about relieving suffering,
allaying fears and improving quality of life – and these are the
main reasons I became a doctor – but having a detailed understanding of medical information and how to communicate health

statistics and risk to patients is not something that's routinely taught in medical school. The interpretation of the benefits a drug offers a patient, in terms of its ability to save their life, is rarely at the forefront of many doctors' minds, and even if it is, seldom is it communicated to patients. In other words, many patients are being prescribed pills and being asked to take them for the rest of their life without being empowered with the information on the chances that those pills will actually save their lives. Simultaneously, they're not being given actionable lifestyle advice to improve their health rapidly and likely improve their quality of life too (something pills for managing many of these conditions very rarely do).

So how much has modern medicine actually contributed to our longevity?

In one fascinating study of 702 adults carried out in the United States in 2014, 80 per cent believed that of the 40-year average increase in life expectancy since the mid 1800s, 32 years were attributed to modern medicine. In fact, nothing could be further from the truth. Best estimates suggest medical care has added only 3.5–5 years to our life expectancy. And the bulk of those years are predominantly due to the antibiotics developed to fight infections; medical treatment for heart disease (especially aspirin); the development of hospital coronary care units; screening and drug treatment of moderate–severe hypertension (high blood pressure); and screening and management of some cancers, especially cervical and colorectal. Insulin for type 1 diabetes and dialysis for kidney failure have also been impactful.

But contrary to what the participants in the survey believed, it is public health interventions that have been responsible for the overwhelming majority of the increases in lifespan – an average of 39 years in 1850 to approximately 79 years now in the US; figures that are not dissimilar to other Western nations, including the UK.

So, what has been responsible for the biggest impact on our increased lifespan over that past 150 years? The ones that top the list include the following:

- *Safer workplaces* – severe injuries and death as a consequence of mining, construction, manufacturing and transportation have dramatically reduced, and due to safer workplace regulations since 1980 there's been a 40 per cent decline in fatal occupational injuries.
- *Better sanitation and safe drinking water* – this was responsible for the control of many infectious diseases that were the big killers in the first half of the twentieth century, such as cholera and typhoid.
- *Better food hygiene and food fortification* – since 1900 this has resulted in a reduction in the spread of contaminated food as well as the identification of necessary trace elements and vitamins (micronutrients) that have been added to foods and have virtually eliminated diseases such rickets and pellagra.
- *Motor vehicle safety improvements* – better motorways and the introduction of seat belts in cars have dramatically reduced death from car accidents.
- *Recognition of tobacco as a health hazard* – in fact, 50 per cent of the decline in death rates from heart disease in the past four decades can be directly attributed to a reduction in the prevalence of smoking.

It's clear that the most important factors that have determined our health and longevity have very little to do with modern medical treatment. As a cardiologist, my early career involved being trained in and specialising in emergency stenting. But I soon realised that rather than saving people from drowning, wouldn't it be much better to stop them falling into the river in the first place? This brings us on to our next chapter, the real pandemic, poor metabolic health.

CHAPTER 3

The Real Pandemic – Poor Metabolic Health

I should warn you that there's quite a lot of science in this chapter, but it's important as it will provide you with essential insight and background to the underlying conditions linked to immunity and, most importantly, how and why the 21-day plan works.

It's the 27th March 2020. The UK and international media reports of a disturbing and increasing death toll from the coronavirus that is now sweeping through hospitals on the east coast of America. I text my friend and colleague, Shahriar, a senior doctor in one of the USA's busiest emergency departments in Brooklyn, New York.

'Are you okay?' I ask.

'Thank you, my friend. I am okay. It's quite surreal here – dire situation. Our already broken healthcare system is on the verge of collapse. There is no better time to pray for us. Please stay safe. Hopefully the situation is better in England.'

'Sending you much love, brother,' I replied.

The scale of the problem

Was Shahriar exaggerating when he referred to America's already broken healthcare system? Sadly not. America spends 18 per cent of its GDP on healthcare – the highest expenditure in the world, equating to an annual spend of approximately $3.5 trillion – yet it ranks 34th in the world for overall health and wellness of its citizens. The latest data suggests the baseline health of most Americans is dire. Just like the UK, more than 60 per cent are overweight or obese, but of greater concern is that 7 out of 8 Americans are affected by poor metabolic health, including a third of those of normal weight (although the data hasn't been collated, it's likely that the figures in the UK are not dissimilar). And this isn't just confined to older age groups. Only 1 in 4 individuals aged between 20 and 40 have optimal metabolic health.

When it comes to demand on healthcare, most of those dollars are spent on community drug and hospital treatment of chronic metabolic diseases, which include cardiovascular disease, type 2 diabetes, high blood pressure and even some common cancers.

As of 2017, 6 out of the top 10 causes of death in the USA can be attributed to sub-optimal metabolic health and 8 out of 10 are predominantly influenced by lifestyle and environment (the conditions in which we are born, grow, live and work). Similarly, the leading causes of death in the UK are also rooted in poor metabolic health.

Modern medicine has an important role to play in treating some of these conditions, offering marginal long-term gains for a few, but extensive evidence reveals that we're prescribing too many pills for lifestyle diseases, resulting in great cost and likely significant harms. Although not included in WHO data, an analysis by one eminent scientist, Professor Peter Goetzche, co-founder of Cochrane (an independent institute of medical research) and published in the *BMJ*, suggests that side effects of prescribed medication are now estimated to be one of the leading causes of death globally after heart disease and cancer, with the elderly the most vulnerable. Given the scale of the problem two well-respected medical journals, the *BMJ* and *JAMA Internal Medicine*, have started campaigns in recent years to reduce the harms of too much medicine. More drugs have not appeared to provide us with the answers to solve the pandemic of the very conditions that collectively make up the bulk of healthcare costs. One chronic metabolic condition whose long-term adverse health impact is particularly disturbing is type 2 diabetes.

Why is type 2 diabetes so devastating?

Type 2 diabetes itself is a disease that affects 400 million globally. South Asians are disproportionately affected, with India now having the highest prevalence of type 2 diabetes in the world. The disease occurs when blood glucose builds up in the blood stream, and usually develops over many years when the body's cells are unable to respond to the hormone insulin. Its dramatic global increase in the past two decades has been directly attributed to the way we live, especially the amount and types of foods we are eating.

Glucose is necessary to provide energy for every cell in our body. It's so vital that even if we're not consuming it in the form of carbohydrate, the body is able to make enough of its own for survival by breaking down fat and protein. Insulin is a hormone produced by the pancreas whose main role is to maintain blood glucose levels within a tight range. When glucose is outside this range for prolonged periods, it starts to cause damage to virtually every organ system in our body. Insulin also plays a role in preventing the breakdown of stored fat to be used as energy; many therefore refer to it as the 'fat-storing' hormone.

Insulin resistance occurs when the cells of the body become resistant to the effects of insulin and thus the pancreas secretes more and more insulin to compensate. Eventually that compensation stops being effective at all and blood glucose rises above the normal range, which then becomes type 2 diabetes. But insulin resistance – or hyperinsulinaemia (chronically-raised insulin) – can be present for many years, even decades, before one is actually diagnosed with type 2 diabetes.

Those with the condition are subject to years of suffering. A study at the University of California looking at those with type 2 diabetes aged between 30 and 75, revealed that almost half suffered from acute and chronic pain similar to patients living with cancer, and a quarter reported fatigue, depression, sleep disturbance and physical and emotional disability:

- 70 per cent of those with type 2 diabetes will also ultimately develop some form of dementia
- 80 per cent of those with type 2 diabetes will eventually die of a thrombotic complication, most commonly heart attack and stroke

In other words, average life expectancy for those with the condition is reduced by 5–15 years. In the UK, it is the single biggest contributor to NHS costs, making up 10% of the annual budget. In the US, its precursor, pre-diabetes, affects 1 in 3 Americans.

The damage from type 2 diabetes at a biological level is partly related to a patient's blood glucose being out of the normal range (see page 13) – the higher the blood glucose the greater the risk of complications. But what is perhaps most concerning about the disease is that the very expensive drug treatment employed to manage it (specifically to keep blood glucose under control) has not only failed to reduce death rates but the side effects are responsible for almost 100,000 visits to US emergency rooms every year. As will also be highlighted in the next chapter, type 2 diabetes itself, especially if poorly controlled, has additionally proven to be associated with a significantly increased risk of death from COVID-19.

Clearly type 2 diabetes is a condition you want to try to avoid at all costs if you can but the good news is that it can also be sent into remission – or at the very least blood glucose can be significantly improved or even kept in the normal range purely from lifestyle changes and therefore without the need for drugs. As many results show, including those of my own patients, significant improvement can happen within weeks – within 21 days, in the majority of cases.

Is obesity the big problem?

For years many doctors and scientists have believed that obesity causes insulin resistance and type 2 diabetes, but the evidence suggests that insulin resistance happens well before one becomes

The twin evils: insulin resistance and chronic inflammation

The underlying process leading to the spectrum of diseases resulting from poor metabolic health, which include type 2 diabetes, is related to insulin resistance and its overlapping evil twin, chronic inflammation. Chronic inflammation can occur either directly as a result of insulin resistance or through a separate mechanism.

Chronically raised insulin, or the body becoming resistant to its effects, are strongly linked to the development of cancer, heart, kidney and liver disease, obesity, Alzheimer's disease and vascular dementia and osteoporosis.

Over 80 per cent of those that develop heart disease have underlying insulin resistance, suggesting that it's the most important risk factor. This is supported by the fact that two thirds of those admitted with heart attacks have metabolic syndrome, the most severe manifestation of insulin resistance.

obese. As I mentioned in the introduction (see page 1), obesity is just the tip of a diet-related-disease iceberg – type 2 diabetes and metabolic syndrome occur in a substantial number of people who are overweight (i.e. not yet diagnosed as obese) and more disturbingly in those with a so-called normal BMI. It is crucial to emphasise this, as many people may be given the illusion of protection that they have a 'healthy weight' based purely on their BMI, and therefore they will not have their metabolic health checked. In fact, nothing could be further from the truth.

Over a ten-year period, research has revealed that those in middle age with poor metabolic health but of a normal weight had a three-fold increased risk of death, heart attack or stroke compared to those who were metabolically healthy with the same weight.

Irrespective of insulin, over time high blood glucose causes damage to practically every major organ in the body – one of the earliest manifestations of insulin resistance occurs in the liver, where excess fat is also stored. All the evidence points to the fact that if we want a long and happy life we should all know our metabolic health status and introduce measures to correct it, regardless of what our weight is. We're all vulnerable.

How does one measure insulin resistance and metabolic health?

The most accurate way is a slightly complicated test that involves injecting both insulin and glucose and taking several measurements over a few hours, but there's a much easier way to measure your own metabolic health. Two measurements can be carried out at home and three will need to be done via a blood test from your GP. At home, you can use a tape measure to determine your waist circumference by measuring it at the level of the belly button. You can also check your blood pressure with a home blood pressure monitor. For the remaining three a simple blood test via your GP will tell you your average blood glucose, triglyceride and HDL-cholesterol levels.

Keeping blood pressure in check

High blood pressure on its own is the single biggest risk factor for death worldwide. It's the most important risk factor for stroke and also a major risk factor for heart attack and kidney disease. According to the World Health Organization there are just over a billion people worldwide who suffer from it, affecting 1 in 4 men and 1 in 5 women.

Blood pressure is best explained as pressure within the major blood vessels of the body. It's determined by the force of blood being pumped from the heart combined with the resistance of the blood flow in the arteries.

What causes high blood pressure?

We learned in medical school that in most cases the cause of high blood pressure (referred to as essential hypertension in medical speak) isn't known, but in reality, what is increasingly being understood is that insulin resistance is linked and may be causal in about 50 per cent of those suffering from high blood pressure. It's also one of the major conditions linked to poor outcomes from COVID-19, perhaps driven by underlying insulin resistance.

Insulin and insulin resistance can raise blood pressure in a number of ways. One is by stimulating the kidneys to retain more sodium, which in turn will result in more retention of water and increase pressure within the blood vessels. Another is by activating the sympathetic nervous system which is responsible for increasing heart rate.

Insulin resistance also interferes with the production of nitric oxide from cells lining the arteries, which is what is involved in dilating and relaxing the arteries. Over time, loss of elasticity and stiffness of the larger blood vessels contributes to increased pressure within these arteries.

Other overlapping and linked factors to high blood pressure include excessive salt intake in a proportion of patients who are salt sensitive, too much alcohol, and smoking. Sugar consumption has also been strongly implicated, and chronic psychological stress and poor sleep may also play a significant role. Again, all these factors are things we have the potential to change ourselves.

One school of thought is that blood pressure increasing is just part of the ageing process, occurring with natural loss of elasticity of the large blood vessels. Insulin resistance also tends to increase with age and although these are both true, they do not tell the full story. Some studies carried out many years ago on rural African tribes with very active lifestyles who were not exposed to processed food had virtually no evidence of the development of high blood pressure, even in older age groups, which suggests that it's not necessarily attributed to advancing years alone and may be entirely preventable given a healthy lifestyle and environmental factors. Our fast-paced way of modern living, accompanied by fast food, makes this more challenging to achieve in Western culture.

If you have high blood pressure you won't necessarily exhibit any symptoms unless it's extremely high, so it's important to get it checked regularly, especially if there's a strong family history of high blood pressure and for everyone aged over 40.

What blood pressure level is normal?

The optimum blood pressure is lower than 120/80mmHg. The first number is known as the systolic blood pressure. This is the maximum pressure in the major arteries that occurs after one heartbeat. The second number is the diastolic pressure. This is the minimum pressure that occurs between two heart beats. The lower level of normal is 90/60mmHg. Above 120/80mmHg the risk of stroke starts to increase. The risk becomes particularly apparent once it's over 140/90 mmHg. Similar to pre-diabetes there's now a definition of pre-hypertension which is when one has readings that fall between these levels.

To summarise:

Pre-hypertension	120/80–139/89mmHg
Mild hypertension	140/90–159/99mmHg
Moderate hypertension	160/100–179/109mmHg
Severe hypertension	any level above 180/110mmHg

The other interesting thing about blood pressure is that sometimes elevated readings will be taken because of acute psychological stress – when seeing the doctor, for example – and may not reflect the average individual's blood pressure. This is known as 'white coat syndrome' and it can elevate blood pressure quite dramatically by even more than 60mmHg. For example, someone whose blood pressure is normally 120mmHg systolic can, in stressful circumstances, go up to 180. One should be in a relaxed state for a good few minutes before blood pressure is checked either by the doctor or with a home blood pressure monitor.

Why not just take a pill?

Let me start by emphasising that medications for high blood pressure have been truly life-saving but they are now hugely over-prescribed and have only a significant benefit in reducing stroke and heart attack in those with average values consistently over 160/100mmHg (moderate hypertension). Unfortunately, the medical community are increasingly beginning to understand that because of too much pharmaceutical industry influence over medical guidelines, many patients in the mild hypertension category are prescribed medication even though evidence reveals that the pill itself will not reduce the risk of heart attack, stroke or death.

In general, blood pressure pills are relatively safe but overall side effects that interfere with quality of life affect about 1 in 10 people taking them and these can often be resolved by stopping or changing the pill. The most common side effects, depending on which drug you're prescribed, are cough, diarrhoea and constipation, light-headedness, erection problems, nausea, headache and fatigue.

Lowering blood pressure through lifestyle

What most doctors either don't know or don't discuss with their patients is that lifestyle changes can have quite dramatic positive effects on one's blood pressure – for example, eating the right foods and cutting out the ones that exacerbate insulin resistance. I have many patients who have managed to reduce their need for medication, even in middle age, and in some cases even come off pills within a few months, just from cutting out sugar and refined carbohydrate foods and eating a Mediterranean-inspired diet combined with taking up regular moderate activity, such as brisk walking. The best part is that unlike a pill, these lifestyle changes have no side effects and usually also improve overall quality of life, something that pills for managing chronic metabolic disease cannot do.

A friend of mine recently asked me for advice for her 63-year-old mother who had been on a blood pressure drug for several years. Following the diet plan outlined in this book she cut out all junk food and high glycaemic carbohydrates and in five weeks she'd not only lost 5kg, to her delight was able to come off the blood pressure pill she'd been taking for years.

Another patient of mine in his eighties, who had suffered from high blood pressure for years, decided to follow my advice and change his lifestyle. He was able to come off his blood pressure pills within a few months. He felt that it was adopting regular meditation that made the most significant impact on his readings.

Both my parents suffered from high blood pressure, both diagnosed in their late forties, and several members of my extended family do too, which would suggest I'm also vulnerable. But I follow my own lifestyle advice and at 42 my blood pressure averages 110/60mmHg. I was also pleasantly surprised to recently find out from a body composition scan that my metabolic age is 29. I'll take that.

The 21-day plan will provide you with all the optimal diet and lifestyle solutions to reduce blood pressure, optimise your metabolic health, reverse metabolic syndrome and maximise your resilience to infection.

CHAPTER 4

How Metabolic Health Affects Our Immunity

When Boris Johnson was admitted to hospital and then intensive care with worsening symptoms of COVID-19 the UK watched in horror. An immediate observation that caused me concern was the prime minister's weight. I knew, as is well established in medical literature that, in general, being obese makes outcomes from infections worse.

What was also clear was that several of his advisors and close colleagues who had also tested positive for the virus (and on the face of it were considerably slimmer), did not appear to suffer any more than mild symptoms and managed by self-isolating at home for two weeks.

A few weeks after the prime minister's recovery and discharge from hospital, I wrote two articles – published in *European Scientist* and in the *Telegraph* – in which I explained how obesity-related conditions, specifically those worse affected by metabolic syndrome, may give you a ten-fold increased risk of dying from the virus.

The main reason the prime minister needed hospital admission was because the virus had affected his lungs to such an extent that he needed oxygen. In most severe cases the lungs get fatigued just to take normal breaths in and out and a mechanical ventilator is required. Sadly with COVID-19, once you get to that state the odds of death are very high – 40%. Fortunately, although it was at one stage touch and go as to whether he would need to go on a ventilator, the prime minister survived and was discharged a few weeks later.

So how does obesity affect the immune system?

Obesity is a measure of body mass index, specifically having a BMI over 30. BMI is calculated by dividing one's weight in kilograms by height in metres squared. For example, if you weigh 70kg and your height is 1.8 metres, you divide 70 by (1.8 x 1.8) = 21.6.

Normal weight is classified as 18–25 and overweight as 25–30.

The limitation of BMI, however, is that it relies solely on weight and height and fails to take account of age, ethnicity, fat distribution and muscle mass.

With ageing there is a decline in muscle mass, especially in those who have poor metabolic health too, whereas waist circumference and percentage body fat tend to increase.

With regard to metabolic health, however, only 1 in 200 who are obese will be metabolically healthy (have all 5 parameters in the normal range, see page 13) so for all intents and purposes obesity is still an important marker of having excess body fat, and therefore highly suggestive of being metabolically unhealthy.

Why is too much body fat bad for the immune system?

Excess body fat has a negative effect on normal immune function in a number of different ways but primarily it's through a process known as chronic inflammation. When we suffer an infection a properly functioning immune and inflammatory response protects us. But when a person has chronic inflammation, their body is constantly under attack from environmental triggers, such as poor diet, smoking and chronic psychological stress which the immune system is constantly responding to and is affected by. Regardless of a person's weight, these factors create a state of chronic inflammation in the body.

When a person has a background of chronic inflammation and is then exposed to a virus, the cells that are responsible for fighting that attack do not function as effectively as they should. These cells, called macrophages, are a type of white blood cell that engulf and digest foreign invaders (antigens), cancer cells and any other cells that are not recognised as healthy. In addition, excess body fat in the abdomen that surrounds the liver, pancreas and even fat underneath the skin (subcutaneous fat) release too much of several pro-inflammatory cytokines. Cytokines are a group of proteins released from immune cells to help regulate the immune response through communication with other cells in the body. It's the 'cytokine storm' from an abnormal immune response that leads to the acute respiratory distress syndrome that causes severe lung injury and death in many of those who are killed by COVID-19. Global data has also revealed that in those under the age of 50 that succumbed, being obese was the biggest risk factor for hospitalisation and death.

In addition, those with excess body fat also have higher levels of leptin, a hormone that is released from fat cells that normally helps control appetite. Those who develop excess weight over time may become resistant to leptin, which hinders their control mechanisms in stopping overeating. Leptin also happens to be another pro-inflammatory hormone.

Obesity also appears to reduce the response to vaccination and increase the risk of viruses mutating. This happens because viruses stay in the body for longer as a result of an inability to produce the full immune response, which allows the virus to replicate for longer and produce a new strain.

Beyond the noble virtue of exercising compassion for fellow human beings there is a strong scientific argument that in order to protect ourselves from new strains of viruses we must all have a stake in ensuring obesity is reduced in the population by supporting policies and efforts to make that happen.

An individual's immune system is the result of a number of factors – and some of them cannot be changed, such as age and genetics, including inherited and acquired conditions that negatively impact on immunity – but many of them such as diet, exercise, weight, alcohol and stress are modifiable.

A number of conditions, especially those related to insulin resistance and metabolic syndrome, are more prevalent in those suffering complications and death from COVID-19. Apart from older age, which is the biggest risk factor, the other conditions are either related to high blood glucose or poor metabolic health driven by excess body fat, and chronic inflammation. Combined they all lead to a sub-optimal immune response. We should therefore think of metabolic disease as a disease of the immune system too.

Viruses and bacteria thrive off high blood sugar

It's well established in medical literature, and something I have witnessed and managed in my career, that diabetes (both type 1 and type 2) is associated with more frequent and more severe infections. For clarity, type 1 diabetes makes up about 10% of all diabetes cases and is not caused by lifestyle but is an autoimmune condition usually starting in young adulthood. For unknown reasons the immune system attacks the pancreas to the point where the amount of insulin being produced becomes so low that it becomes incompatible with life. Patients with type 1 always need administered insulin as a drug for life.

Just as diabetes affects many organs, infections also affect many organs in patients with diabetes. It's difficult to know why exactly those with type 1 diabetes have more risk of infectious complications but it could be the combination of both high levels of administered insulin combined with high blood sugar being particularly lethal when it comes to the immune system. If you remember from the previous chapter even excess insulin naturally produced by the body before average blood glucose levels become abnormal has a pro-inflammatory effect.

In the UK, without specifying differences in blood glucose, it was noted that compared to non-diabetics those with type 2 diabetes who contracted coronavirus had a twofold increased risk in death and those with type 1 diabetes had a 3.5 times increase.

The same applies to high blood glucose independently. One study in China revealed that type 2 diabetics admitted to hospital with poor glucose control had a 10-fold increased risk of death in comparison with those with better glucose control.

Given all this data it would be wise to significantly minimise and in the most vulnerable groups avoid altogether foods that are going to raise blood glucose above the normal range. In chapter 6 I'll highlight which types of food these are (see page 49). I'll also explain how for those with type 2 diabetes, blood glucose alone can be improved within just a few days of changing a person's diet and can even be sent into remission within 28 days in a significant proportion. As for those with type 1 diabetes, much better control of average blood glucose and the requirement for less insulin is also very achievable from optimising the types of food we eat.

Ageing and immunity

We cannot ignore the impact of ageing on immunity, especially as with coronavirus it's the biggest risk factor by far for death. For example, those aged over 65 account for 80 per cent of hospitalisation compared to those under 65, and are 23 times more likely to die. However, it's important to note that the overwhelming majority of those that died from COVID-19 in older age groups had at least one underlying condition, predominantly rooted in poor metabolic health. For example, in Italy the average age of death was 81, and those who died had at least two underlying conditions including heart disease, high blood pressure and cancer.

Ageing in general is associated with a decline in the immune system's ability to undertake four specific tasks in responding to an external pathogen:

1. Recognise
2. Alert
3. Destroy
4. Clear

Some over the age of 100 have, however, been able to survive COVID-19, which is most likely due to a combination of good metabolic health and some genetic protection.

But as you've already probably guessed, the major related issues affecting the elderly, not including its link to COVID-19, are lifestyle related, with the overwhelming majority rooted in poor metabolic health. The main conditions are coronary heart disease, diabetes, chronic obstructive lung disease (almost exclusively smoking related), heart failure, stroke, cancer, depression, anxiety and dementia.

And an older population with chronic disease doesn't just bring suffering to millions of individuals and their families, it's also a huge stress to the NHS and social care. In the UK a fifth of the population is over 60 and older people account for the largest single group of patients using the NHS. They account for 60% of the £16.1 billion social care expenditure by local authorities and 40% of all hospital bed stays. These statistics paint a heart-breaking picture – it shouldn't be this way and we can do something about it.

For example, injury due to falls is the leading cause of death in those aged over 75. This is fuelled by poor nutrition combined with lack of exercise. Disturbingly only 17% of men and 13% of women aged 65–74 take enough exercise to meet international guidelines of 30 minutes of moderate exercise at least 5 days a week. For those over 75, this reduces to 8% of men and 3% of women. Just like obesity, vaccine effectiveness for influenza is markedly reduced in older age groups but several studies have revealed that exercise can significantly increase the antibody response to influenza vaccine.

According to the charity Age UK, 'Healthy ageing may be considered as the promotion of healthy living and the prevention and management of illness and disability associated with ageing. Ageing can be thought of as an accumulation of changes over the life course that increases frailty. If we can design and execute effective interventions to prevent or delay the onset of chronic disease and increase healthy life expectancy, there will be social, economic, and health dividends for us all.'

It's therefore time to change the narrative from how an ageing population is a burden on healthcare and society to how an *unhealthy* ageing population is – and it's almost entirely preventable.

CASE STUDY: No one should have to suffer like my mother

One of the most harrowing personal examples of how lifestyle factors affecting metabolic health can rip a family apart is my own experience of the tragic premature death of my own mother.

In November 2018, aged 68, Dr Anisha Malhotra was admitted to hospital with vomiting and excruciating back pain, which even high doses of morphine could only partially relieve. Diagnosed with an infection in her spine, discitis, the only treatment was with intravenous antibiotics. But despite the most potent anti-microbial agents her body, already extremely frail from years of gradual decline, was so overwhelmed by the stress of the infection that she was unable to recover. To make the situation worse, despite having no known heart problems she suffered a heart attack 10 days before she eventually passed away.

Having to witness the suffering and indescribable pain my mother went through still brings me to tears when I think about it. No one should have to go through it and no friend or family member should have to witness it. For the last three years of her life, because of mobility problems due to a combination of severe osteoarthritis and rheumatoid arthritis my mum was also completely dependent on my father who was her main carer. In the six months prior to her final hospital stay she was admitted twice with spontaneous osteoporotic fractures of the bones of her pelvis.

With what I now know about the impact of nutrition and lifestyle on health, I realise that this was entirely avoidable.

For most of her adult life my mum was a vegetarian and significantly overweight, with a BMI of 30. Growing up I witnessed her regular consumption of snack foods – biscuits, crisps and chocolates. I still have a vivid memory of her only meal on her weekly fast day (as a devout Hindu) consisting of a single chapati and what can only be described as a mountain of table sugar.

Although she never suffered from type 2 diabetes, it's likely that her insulin levels were high and, combined with her excess body fat, manifested itself as high blood pressure for which she required medication in her forties. Then at the age of 54 she suffered a brain haemorrhage from which she was lucky to survive. Despite making a full recovery and taking up going to the gym three times a week and even learning to swim in her mid-fifties, her diet and weight didn't change much and over the next 10 years there began a gradual deterioration in her mobility. Obesity-related osteoarthritis led to severe degeneration of her spine, forcing her to take early retirement from her job as a GP, and the chronic joint pain she suffered resulted in her popping painkillers like Smarties.

Prior to my mum's final hospital admission, her loss of muscle mass meant that her BMI had dropped to 20, so obesity wouldn't even have factored into her death when in fact it was at the root of all her problems.

My mum's case is sadly not an isolated anecdote but reflects much of the evidence on the type of diet many Indians follow, including those who are vegetarian. It's instructive to note that India, with more vegetarians and vegans than all other countries combined, is the type 2 diabetes capital of the world. In the past 50 years, to coincide with rocketing prevalence of type 2 diabetes the subcontinent has seen increases of processed wheat, sugar and industrial seed oils (also known as vegetable oils), which have overtaken animal fats (such as butter and ghee) as a percentage of calories.

Protein deficiency is an increasing problem in the elderly but seems to be an even bigger problem amongst Indians. The Indian Dietetic Association recently reported that 84% of Indians were protein deficient. Calorie for calorie meat is more nutrient dense and proteinaceous than vegetables.

Loss of muscle mass is a natural part of the ageing process but it can be significantly mitigated with the right diet (including getting enough protein) and keeping active. This is not just good for the immune system and metabolic health but reduces the risk of falls and bone fractures. Remember from the previous chapter the single biggest cause of mortality in those over 75 is falls.

CHAPTER 5

Why Our Diet Might Be Making Us Ill

Eighty per cent of chronic disease is attributable to lifestyle and linked environmental factors. And within the lifestyle hierarchy, poor diet is the most important contributor, now responsible for more disease and death than physical inactivity, smoking and alcohol combined. Global deaths from sub-optimal nutrition are currently estimated to be at 11 million per year.

So what constitutes poor diet exactly?

According to the most recent Lancet study, there are a number of specific dietary factors which either through excessive or inadequate intake contribute to chronic metabolic diseases. In other words, a poor diet is best described as not getting all the important nutrients for good health from food while eating the kind of products that over time will make you fat and unwell. The major dietary culprits include excessive salt, a diet low in whole fruit and vegetables, inadequate intake of nuts and seeds, not enough omega 3 fats, not enough fibre, too much sugar, and a high intake of processed meat.

Directly linked to poor diet is our overconsumption of ultra-processed food and drink, which has displaced the consumption of whole nutritious food. As I'll explain below, ultra-processed foods and drinks are now the number one enemy in the Western diet, making up more than a staggering 50% of calories consumed on average in the UK. In summary, ultra-processed food and drink is essentially any industrial formulation (a packaged product) with five or more ingredients usually containing sugar, unhealthy oils and salt, and which are lacking in fibre, vitamins and minerals. Examples of typical ultra-processed products include: carbonated drinks; ice-cream and confectionery; mass-produced packaged breads and buns; margarines and spreads; breakfast 'cereals', 'fruit' yoghurts; and 'health' and 'slimming' products, to name just a few.

Because these foods are deliberately designed by the food industry to be cheap and hyperpalatable, they also encourage overconsumption, are mildly addictive and likely to stimulate appetite. In the extreme they're either being eaten instead of what you should be consuming, making you nutritionally deficient and sick, or being eaten on top of what you should be eating, making you fat and sick at the same time. Obesity researcher Dr Zoe Harcombe refers to these products as 'fake food' and I agree. Numerous published studies now link their consumption with adverse health outcomes, independent of weight gain. But as you have already learned when it comes to BMI there's no such thing as a healthy weight, only a healthy person and that means optimum metabolic health.

Even much of the bread we buy regularly in the UK is ultra-processed. There are often more than a dozen ingredients in a typical supermarket loaf, including additives and preservatives –

even the ones labelled as 'healthy brown bread'. There's some recent data suggesting that the additives themselves raise basal levels of insulin independently of the type of food being consumed and studies on mice reveal that additives have an adverse effect on the gut microbiome, which in itself contributes to chronic inflammation. As the maxim goes, if your granny wouldn't recognise some of the ingredients, don't eat it!

With regard to weight gain, a fascinating landmark randomised controlled study was carried out and published in 2019 by US-based pioneering obesity researcher Dr Kevin Hall. The aim of the research trial was to see what would happen when comparing two diets matched for presented calories in addition to sugar, fibre, fat and total macronutrients. One diet contained only unprocessed whole food and the other was ultra-processed. Each of the 20 weight-stable participants could eat as much as they liked and were allowed to eat until fullness. Over a two-week period the diet of ultra-processed food resulted in an extra 500 calories a day being consumed and a 1kg weight gain. And the unprocessed food diet, which resulted in 500 calories less being consumed, resulted in a 1kg weight loss.

As we've learned in previous chapters, chronic low-grade inflammation is also triggered by excess body fat and is an underlying component of poor metabolic health and a poorly functioning immune system. But what is little known is that Western diet foods themselves also have pro-inflammatory effects.

There are numerous studies in published medical literature which reveal that even in the short term, consuming ultra-processed foods and drinks can increase markers of chronic inflammation independently of body weight. For example, just a few weeks of consuming a daily diet of fast food containing trans-fats raises insulin, visceral fat and blood markers of inflammation. The consumption of one sugary drink per day in healthy young men increases markers of insulin resistance and an important marker of chronic inflammation within 21 days.

What's so bad about sugar?

Sugar has no nutritional value whatsoever and optimum consumption for health is zero. It's the number one dietary factor driving tooth decay, chronic pain and hospital admissions in young children.

When it comes to metabolic syndrome it's one of the main dietary culprits when consumed in excess. The World Health Organization now recommends an ideal maximum limit per day of no more than six teaspoons in total, which includes all added sugar in foods, sugar in fruit juice, smoothies, honey and syrups. The average UK citizen is still consuming at least two to three times the maximum recommended limit.

One should really view these foods as directly toxic to the body, certainly when consumed on a daily basis. Ditching ultra-processed food and drink is a good place to start in an effort to improve metabolic health and most likely immune resilience, but it's equally important not to ignore, particularly if you're overweight, obese or metabolically unhealthy, the other big culprits linked to the increasing burden of chronic disease – low quality carbohydrates.

Understanding carbohydrates and the glycaemic index

Low-quality carbohydrates are most easily defined as carbohydrates that lack fibre and they are often high glycaemic index carbohydrates. The glycaemic index (GI) is a figure calculated by the relative rise in glucose in the blood after consuming a food, specifically carbohydrates. GI values are usually divided into three categories:

LOW GI: 1–55
MEDIUM GI: 56–69
HIGH GI: 70 and above

Low-quality carbohydrates have the greatest impact on blood glucose and insulin responses after consumption, which is what we want to avoid as much as possible for the purposes of our metabolic health. Regular consumption results in chronic high blood glucose which will lead to an increase in the production of inflammatory markers. Not surprisingly there's a clear association with the high consumption of these foods and the development of type 2 diabetes, heart disease and obesity.

Foods that are classified as low-quality carbohydrates are all types of bread, white rice, pasta, added sugar, potatoes, and fruit juice. You may be surprised about potatoes. Although potatoes contain vitamin C, potassium and some fibre, they're predominantly composed of starch with a high glycaemic index. Some recent studies have revealed that a higher intake of potatoes in all forms (baked, boiled, mashed, and French fries) is associated with weight gain, type 2 diabetes and the development of high blood pressure.

High-quality carbohydrates, such as whole fruit and non-starchy vegetables (such as green beans, spinach, cabbage, broccoli and cauliflower); pulses and legumes, such as peas, beans and lentils; and whole grains, such as wheat berries, oats and quinoa tend to be low and medium glycaemic index foods. It's especially important if you have excess body fat, type 2 diabetes, metabolic syndrome (80% of the UK population) or want to achieve optimal metabolic health, to consume carbohydrates that are predominantly low glycaemic index.

So now that you know the major issue in what to avoid eating and why, let's move on to the most beneficial foods for metabolic health that you should be eating instead.

CHAPTER 6
Food is Medicine

'It's time we realise that food is a form of healthcare and promote a proper human dietary lifestyle'

—*Dr Ravi Kamepalli, infectious diseases and obesity physician*

For decades much of the mainstream health mantra has been to maintain a healthy weight and count calories which as you've now discovered is both wrong and misguided. A healthy weight doesn't exist, at least in terms of metabolic health, and when it comes to calories it's the quality of calories that influences nutritional value, affects inflammation and influences metabolic health.

So can what we eat significantly improve risk factors for disease and help prevent longer-term harms of suffering from a heart attack, stroke or death? My own clinical experience supported by up-to-date published evidence answers this question with an emphatic yes.

Towards the middle of the twentieth century, when heart disease was rapidly increasing in countries such as the USA and the UK, traditional Mediterranean populations had a much lower incidence of heart disease. Although it's likely that was due to a combination of lifestyle factors, published studies suggest that the benefits were mostly linked to their diet, more specifically, consuming extra virgin olive oil as their main source of fat, eating an abundance of whole fruits and vegetables, oily fish, nuts and seeds and dairy from cheese and yoghurt.

Although there are variations between the Mediterranean countries of Greece, Italy and Spain, Mediterranean diets do tend to be high in omega-3 fats, oleic acid, fibre and antioxidants.

Diet does save lives

The Lyon Heart study published in the Lancet in 2001 was a randomised trial in which 605 patients who had survived a heart attack were prescribed either a Mediterranean diet or a standard low-fat American Heart Association (AHA) diet. After four years there was a quite astonishing reduction in rates of heart attack, cancer and death in those patients following the Mediterranean diet compared to the AHA diet. Death occurred in 34 of 303 (8.0%) in those following the AHA diet plan versus only 14 out of 302 (4.6%) in those following the Mediterranean diet. There were 17 new cancers in those on the AHA diet (8.2%) versus only 7 (2.3%) in the Mediterranean diet group. Finally, there were 33 (8.2%) non-fatal heart attacks in the AHA group versus 8 (2.6%) in the Mediterranean diet group.

When we break this information down, for every 18 people prescribed the Mediterranean diet, one heart attack was prevented compared to those following the standard so-called heart-healthy low-fat American Heart Association diet.

The PREDIMED study published in *the New England Journal of Medicine* in 2013 was a randomised trial involving over 5000 participants who were considered at high risk of developing heart disease in the future. Two groups were asked to follow a Mediterranean diet but one was specifically asked to consume at least 4 tablespoons of extra virgin olive oil (EVOO) every day and the other a handful of tree nuts (almonds, walnuts or hazelnuts). The comparison group was a lower fat Mediterranean diet. After almost five years the ones on the Mediterranean diet supplemented with EVOO or nuts experienced fewer strokes.

What's interesting about both PREDIMED and Lyon is that the benefits in reduction of heart attack and stroke occurred independently of any reduction in cholesterol or weight loss. The most likely explanation is that the anti-inflammatory components of the dietary patterns reduced risk of developing heart disease and stroke.

The elements in the diet that are thought to have led to the changes were the anti-inflammatory polyphenols (organic chemicals) and omega-3 fatty acids found in fruit and vegetables, oily fish, nuts and extra virgin olive oil, which are the basis of a traditional Mediterranean diet.

It's also important to be aware that both comparison diet plans in the Lyon and PREDIMED studies were still considered to be healthy by modern standards. It's likely that the benefits of the Mediterranean diet, and that with added EVOO, would be much greater if compared to the type of diet laden with ultra-processed food that many of us are eating today.

On a population level, analysis by two eminent nutrition and public health scientists, Dariush Mozaffarian and Simon Capewell, suggest that even modest shifts in dietary patterns (such as eating more whole fruit and vegetables, seafood and nuts, for example) could halve the number of deaths from heart attack and stroke globally within a year – taking them from 20 million to 10 million.

But what about metabolic health and metabolic syndrome?

Risk factors for metabolic health and metabolic syndrome can reverse within 21 days of diet and lifestyle changes even independent of weight loss. Comparing various levels of carbohydrate restriction, a 28-day trial of 15 obese patients with metabolic syndrome revealed more than 50% were able to reverse a diagnosis of metabolic syndrome just by eliminating sugar and starchy foods from their diet. This occurred without any change in weight. The authors tested this hypothesis on purpose to reveal what changes in diet can do to metabolic markers of risk without weight loss. They concluded that if weight had been lost then the effect would have likely been much greater.

A previous diet and exercise study carried out by researchers at the University of California involving 31 participants also revealed reversal of metabolic syndrome in 50 per cent of those that followed a low-fat, high-fibre diet combined with 45–60 minutes of moderate-intensity exercise per day. Markers of insulin resistance improved but again there was no correlation with weight loss, suggesting an independent benefit on metabolic health. Similar rapid improvements in markers of metabolic health with reversal of metabolic syndrome in all participants were observed in a trial involving 7 obese children following a diet and exercise programme within 21 days.

Dietary patterns with high fibre intake are linked to keeping body fat levels down, helping to keep blood glucose in a normal range, linked to reduced risk of developing type 2 diabetes and reducing the risk of colon cancer.

My colleague Professor Robert Lustig revealed that despite keeping calories the same (including those from carbohydrates), reduction in sugar (specifically fructose) from 28% of calories to 10% in 43 obese children had a remarkable impact on markers of metabolic syndrome independent of weight loss. There was a 5mmHg drop in blood pressure, and a 33-point drop in triglycerides and also significant drops in blood glucose and fasting insulin.

The children reported that they noticed they felt less hungry. Again, what's consistent is that there was no ultra-processed food, as well as minimal to zero sugar and other low-quality carbohydrates in these trials. The message is clear. Dietary changes are rapid and substantial

Food as medicine for diabetes

In the past few years there's been great interest in the 'reversal' of type 2 diabetes. We were taught in medical school that this is a chronic progressive, irreversible condition, but increasing evidence reveals that that assertion is false.

Following publication of my first book, *The Pioppi Diet*, a 21-day lifestyle plan, an experiment was carried out with my guidance by a doctor for a Dutch television programme. Three randomly selected volunteers tested my claim that the diet could improve weight and metabolic health within 21 days without counting calories. Not surprisingly all the participants were sceptical when they started but the elation and emotion they all experienced when they were given their results after strictly following the plan for 21 days still gives me goose bumps. One lady who had struggled with her weight for years effortlessly lost 10kg and felt better both mentally and physically. The second middle-aged gentleman who had recently been diagnosed with heart disease and high blood pressure was able to come off one of his blood pressure pills. The third man had the most extraordinary results of all. Ferdy, a train driver in his sixties, had been diagnosed with type 2 diabetes more than ten years previously. His blood glucose was creeping up and he was needing increasing doses of medication. He had just been told by his doctor that the next step was to take insulin, which could impact his ability to continue working as a train driver because of the effect of low blood sugar on his alertness. Within 21 days of cutting out starch and sugar and adopting a Mediterranean-inspired diet he'd come off all his medication and sent his type 2 diabetes into remission. It's been two years since then and he's still in remission. More importantly he feels his quality of life is significantly better.

Now, three years since *The Pioppi Diet* was published, a lot more data has gathered to support it. Far from being an isolated anecdote, what happened to Ferdy is increasingly reflected in large trials and medical practice. NHS GP Dr David Unwin has led pioneering work in the management of type 2 diabetes. By adopting a similar approach in his own practice, he's managed to sustain remission over 30 months in 49.9% (82 out of 166) patients through advising a real-food low-carb diet. This has also resulted in cost savings from diabetes medicine of tens of thousands of pounds per year (in his practice).

Dr Campbell Murdoch, a GP who focuses on metabolic health and a Royal College of General Practitioners clinical adviser, follows a similar approach to David Unwin and informed me that with his own type 2 diabetes patients, within just two days of them quitting starchy and sugary foods he's seen an improvement in blood glucose levels. Remember that poorly controlled blood glucose in type 2 diabetes patients is also a risk factor for increased mortality from infection, which was again more recently highlighted in COVID-19.

Lifestyle first

Let's not completely discount modern medicines, which have achieved some remarkable things in managing acute conditions, such as aspirin for heart attacks or antibiotics for life-threatening bacterial infections. But, as previously outlined, for the conditions rooted in poor metabolic health, which exert the greatest demand on healthcare, there's little evidence that drugs increase lifespan for the overall majority, and can also come with side effects.

A lifestyle approach, which aims to identify the root causes, should be at the forefront of managing these chronic metabolic conditions, with the back-up of modern medicine. But this also means that doctors and patients should be having a more honest and informed discussion about what the true benefits and potential harms are of different drug treatments and what feasible lifestyle changes could be effectively made in keeping with the patient's personal preferences and values. It's what's called shared decision-making. In the 21-day plan I hope to show you just how manageable and effective simple changes to lifestyle can be.

CHAPTER 7

Do I Need to Take Supplements?

'What is clear is that conditions of nutrient deficiency impair the functioning of the immune system and increase susceptibility to infection.'

—McAuliffe S, Ray S, Fallon E et al. 'Dietary micronutrients in the wake of COVID-19: an appraisal of evidence with a focus on high risk-risk groups and preventative healthcare', BMJ Nutrition Prevention and Health 2020

The vitamin industry is a huge business, with the global dietary supplements market size estimated at over $120 billion per year. And yet despite this, studies suggest that those who take supplements are no more likely to live longer than those who don't.

By following a varied diet of whole foods from both plant and animal sources, i.e. eating a variety of vegetables, whole fruits, berries, nuts, seeds, pulses, dairy, oily fish and some meat, most people can obtain all the essential vitamins and micronutrients they need for health.

When it comes to immunity, a number of vitamins (A, B6, B12, folate, C, D and E) and trace elements (zinc, copper, selenium, iron) are essential for optimising and supporting immune function, therefore we should be making sure we eat a variety of foods that contain them. The table below illustrates the best whole food sources of these vitamins and the overwhelming majority of adults can obtain these from a varied diet without the need for supplementation. There are of course exceptions and people who, for various reasons, can't get enough nutrients from their diet, an example being vegans who cannot get vitamin B12 from their diet (it is only available in animal products) and therefore need to supplement.

Having said that we can get all the vitamins we need from our diet, it would be unscientific to completely disregard the use of supplements. Two important vitamins that help support normal immune function deserve a special mention where the evidence suggests that some people may well benefit from supplementation, without any significant risk of harm. Those are vitamin C and vitamin D.

Vitamin C

Vitamin C has a role in many aspects of normal immune function including killing bacteria and antibody production. Foods typically high in vitamin C include oranges, red and green peppers, strawberries and broccoli.

In terms of the common cold, research revealed that extra doses don't stop you getting it but it does reduce both the severity and duration of colds in both children and adults. The standard minimum recommended daily amount from our diet (RDA) is 100mg/day. As there are no significant harms from taking a high dose of vitamin C for short periods of time – a few days to weeks – and the most commonly reported side effect is stomach upset, I recommend my patients take high doses, 1–3g per day (10–30 times the RDA), if and when they feel run down, or more vulnerable to catching a cold from a particularly bad night's rest, or during major travel such as a flight (in this instance I'll take a high dose, such as 1g, the day before, the day of, and for a few days after travelling). I've suffered some of the nastiest bouts of colds within a few days of a flight and we know that the circumstances on aeroplanes – recirculated air and being cooped up with other passengers who may have coughs or colds – are an environment highly conducive to viral transmission.

Vitamin D

Vitamin D has a complex and very important role in the immune system and functions as a hormone in most cells of the body.

The most important source of vitamin D is sun exposure. As a general rule of thumb this means being out in the sun for at least 10 minutes per day exposing forearms, hands and lower legs without sunscreen during the summer months from late March until the end of September. After sun exposure, the most important food sources of vitamin D are oily fish, egg yolks and liver, but these are not usually enough to provide us with the levels we need, so if you find it difficult to meet your needs through these means, then you'll need to take a supplement, at least during the winter months. Unless you have your levels checked by a doctor, you won't know whether you need to supplement all year round, but the NHS website recommends taking 10 micrograms of vitamin D per day through the winter months.

Important dietary sources of nutrients that support the immune system

Nutrient	Good dietary sources
Vitamin A	Milk and cheese; eggs, liver, oily fish; dark green and orange vegetables, including carrots, sweet potatoes, pumpkin, squash kale, spinach, broccoli; orange fruits, such as apricots, peaches, papaya, mango and cantaloupe melon
Vitamin B6	Fish, poultry, meat, eggs, oats, green and leafy vegetables (such as spinach, kale and cabbage), fruits, soya
Vitamin B12	Fish, meat, some shellfish, milk, cheese, eggs
Folate	Broccoli, Brussels sprouts, green leafy vegetables, peas, chickpeas
Vitamin C	Oranges, lemons, red and green peppers, strawberries, blackcurrants, kiwi, Brussels sprouts, potatoes
Vitamin D	Oily fish, liver, egg yolks, mushrooms

Vitamin E	Extra virgin olive oil, nuts and seeds
Zinc	Shellfish (especially oysters), meat, cheese, seeds
Selenium	Fish, shellfish, meat, eggs, Brazil nuts
Iron	Meat, liver, beans, nuts, dried fruit (e.g. raisins, dates and apricots), most dark green leafy vegetables, such as spinach and kale
Copper	Shellfish, nuts, liver, some vegetables
Essential amino acids	Meat, poultry, fish, eggs, milk and cheese, soya, nuts and seeds, pulses
Essential fatty acids	Nuts and seeds
Long chain omega-3 fatty acids (EPA and DHA)	Oily fish

Source: adapted from 'Nutrition, immunity and COVID-19', BMJ Nutrition Prevention And Health, Philip C. Calder

There's been a lot of publicity around the link between vitamin D deficiency and worse outcomes from coronavirus. A study from Indonesia revealed a ten-fold difference in death rates between those with the lowest levels versus those with normal levels. But giving supplementation to those admitted to intensive care revealed no benefit – it may be too late by then. It's therefore better to just ensure your vitamin D levels are always optimised.

Vitamin D deficiency is very common in the population especially in those from BAME (Black and Minority Ethnic) backgrounds who require more sun exposure than those with lighter skin to generate enough vitamin D in the body. Given that deficient or severely deficient vitamin D levels currently affect the majority of those from BAME backgrounds in the UK, my own view is that until proven otherwise presume you're deficient and take a supplement, if BAME, and if Caucasian ensure to take 10 micrograms per day through the winter months.

In summary, you can get all the nutrients you need from diet for normal immune function, except for vitamin D for which you'll need enough sunshine. Given modern living, if this is not feasible or if you have particular dietary preferences (such as following a vegan diet) then you may need to take a supplement. When it comes to vitamin C the jury is out on true benefits but as there's no real demonstrable harm and it may do you some good in certain situations, it's not unreasonable to top up with a supplement from time to time, such as in the examples outlined above.

CHAPTER 8

Exercise is a Wonder Drug

'I believe that if physical activity was a drug it would be classed as a wonder drug, which is why I would encourage everyone to get up and be active'.

—Professor Dame Sue Bailey

Years ago while working as a junior doctor I suffered the worst bout of flu I could ever have imagined. With a high fever and a cough, it took me a week before I was able to get out of bed and six weeks before I felt I had my normal strength and energy. Retrospectively I ascertained that there were three things before I became sick that made what should have been a relatively mild illness much more debilitating.

Firstly, I was particularly stressed that week which also impacted my sleep. To cope I ended up eating snack foods like chocolate bars, biscuits and crisps (this was well before I had become enlightened about how bad such foods were for my health). At one stage I calculated that I was easily consuming up to 40 teaspoons of added sugar per day – now it's close to zero. But the icing on the immunity-destroying cake was that I over-trained a couple of days before my symptoms appeared. Thinking about reducing my stress and feeling guilty because of gorging on junk food that week, I decided I would run at a high intensity for an hour as opposed to my usual 30-minute jog.

What I didn't realise at the time was that my behaviour was significantly ramping up the stress hormones in my body, namely adrenaline and cortisol, which are known to biologically supress the immune system. This didn't just put me more at risk of catching an infection; it meant that my symptoms would be more severe. Sports science research has revealed that although moderate exercise naturally optimises immune function and should be actively encouraged, overdoing it – especially without adequate nutrition, sleep and recovery – has the opposite effect, particularly for respiratory infections. One study demonstrated that elite athletes were twice as likely to develop upper respiratory tract infections than sedentary individuals and four times more likely than recreational athletes. In other words when it comes to immunity, regular exercise in moderation is key.

The immune system is very responsive to physical activity. On a biological level, even a single bout of moderate to vigorous exercise enhances the immune system's ability to function and fight infection more effectively. Over time, with daily exercise, these effects build up to strengthen immune defence activity by positively influencing the function of a number of cells. In addition, moderate activity produces anti-inflammatory cytokines and improves metabolic health.

Conversely, overdoing doing it with bouts of prolonged exercise, especially if the individual is not well rested or nourished, can have short-term negative effects on immune function, increasing inflammation, muscle damage and risk of illness.

How much should we be exercising each week to maintain optimum health and a well-functioning immune system?

The Chief Medical Officer's guidelines for adults state that we should be engaging in at least 150 minutes of moderate activity per week and/or 75 minutes of vigorous-intensity activity per week, as well as some form of strength-building exercise on at least two days per week.

Moderate activity includes brisk walking, swimming or cycling. This can be broken up into 30 minutes 5 times per week or 22 minutes every day. I've given advice on how your heart rate can tell you you're in the moderate activity zone in the 21-day plan (see page 80) but as a guide, for moderate activity it is that you feel a bit out of breath but able to talk.

With vigorous-intensity activity you should be breathing much faster and find it difficult to talk. Examples include running, climbing the stairs or playing tennis or football.

Building strength to keep muscles, joints and bones strong can be done through weight lifting at the gym, carrying heavy bags or yoga.

For adults aged over 60, it's really important to encourage participation in an activity that improves balance at least twice a week. Dancing, bowling and tai chi are good examples.

Contrary to popular belief, when it comes to longevity, there is no evidence to suggest that the more exercise you do the longer you will live (after doing regular moderate activity). For example, elite athletes don't live any longer than say golfers or cricketers. Of course, there will be some individual variation; for example, the genetics of South Asians give rise to lower cardiorespiratory fitness and so they appear to need significantly more activity per week (233 minutes of moderate activity) to achieve the same cardiometabolic benefits as a white European carrying out 150 minutes per week.

The benefits of regular moderate activity on metabolic health and many chronic diseases are summarised below in a report produced by the Academy of Medical Royal Colleges that I co-authored in 2015, titled 'Exercise – the miracle cure'. Doing 30 minutes of moderate exercise 5 times a week reduces the risk of developing cardiovascular disease, type 2 diabetes, dementia and some cancers by at least 30%.

But like improving metabolic health through lifestyle it's not just about the potential long- and short-term health gains, it's about quality of life too. We know that regular activity helps improve those suffering from mild depression, for example, but for virtually every one of my patients and friends I speak to they feel more alert, relaxed and happier in general during and after doing some form of activity that generates a bit of sweat.

The more pressing major issue, however, is that 40% of adults in the UK are not managing to get in the recommended 30 minutes per day, 5 times per week and only 1 in 3 over the age of 65 are doing so, with even worsening levels with increasing age.

The reasons for this are multi-factored and include lack of knowledge, time, motivation, being empowered or supported by friends and a physical environment that facilitates the change.

But just like diet, exercise is not part of routine prescription in modern medical practice. Not because doctors don't know exercise is good for you but they may not have the more precise knowledge of how much and at what intensity and the precise benefits to pass on easily. Surveys also reveal that many doctors feel there's not enough time to discuss lifestyle during a short consultation of 10 minutes per patient. But it can be done through gaining knowledge and confidence to have these discussions as I have regularly done through my NHS clinics.

What I also tell my patients is that if your diet is poor then you're much less likely to be maximising the benefits of exercise. When it comes to markers of metabolic health the power of exercise is dwarfed by the power of dietary changes.

One of the most published and eminent sports scientists in the world, Professor Timothy Noakes, says that if you have to exercise to keep your weight down then your diet is wrong.

In the 21-day plan I'll guide you in understanding exactly how to measure the right level of exercise for the maximum health benefits – not too little and not too much.

CHAPTER 9
Managing Our Stress Levels

When a 49-year-old man called Iqbal came to see me for a 'heart check' last year his story fascinated me. Four years earlier he'd survived a heart attack and received a single stent to a blocked artery through emergency angioplasty. But why did he have a heart attack so young? He told me that over the previous 15 years his lifestyle was the very worst it could be. As a successful but highly stressed executive his diet was full of ultra-processed foods and low-quality carbohydrates. He was also smoking 30 cigarettes per day, was largely sedentary, and had been taking over 100 international flights a year. He had developed mildly raised blood pressure, pre-diabetes and had increased his waist circumference but wasn't obese. By 2015 a heart attack changed his life forever.

Struggling with mild depression and finding it difficult to change his lifestyle he'd been referred by a psychiatrist to a cardiac specialist nurse and stress reduction expert Sherezade Ruano. Sherezade is unique and highly effective in her approach. Following a combination of mindfulness techniques and gentle yoga, in just a few weeks Iqbal felt better than he had in 20 years, as if a huge weight had been lifted off his shoulders. Sherezade also prescribed him a diet and exercise plan for life that he found easy to follow, he managed to quit smoking and he reversed his metabolic syndrome within weeks. 'She completely transformed my life,' he told me. 'I don't think I could have done any of this without her help.' Now mindfulness meditation is just an automatic part of his daily routine. When he came to me to be checked five years later, I repeated all his blood tests and at his request organised a special heart scan which revealed no progression or new areas of heart disease.

The experience of stress is very subjective but invariably all the patients who consult me who have suffered a heart attack cite stress as a significant contributing factor, especially those under 60. When I ask them to give an average score from zero to ten of their stress levels in the months to years leading up to the heart attack it's invariably above seven. We know that a stressful life also makes one more likely to succumb to an unhealthy lifestyle, but research has also revealed that lowering stress has an independent effect over diet and exercise, reducing the progression of the build-up of blockages in heart arteries and even potentially reversing those narrowings. So just adhering to a healthy diet and moderate regular exercise isn't enough, we need to be proactive about how to keep our stress levels in check too. Stress increases markers of inflammation in the blood, which studies have shown to be predictive of the development of heart disease.

What Iqbal had effectively done was help to reverse his metabolic syndrome by reducing the stress that was at the root of his poor lifestyle behaviours. He did this by learning to practise mindfulness but there are many different ways to manage stress and individuals will differ in what works for them. For some, it will be breathing deeply for 10–20 minutes first thing in the morning; for others it might be joining a yoga or Pilates class. Even making it a habit to be more proactive through social interaction can reap huge benefits.

Chronic stress plays a significant role in the development of most, if not all, chronic metabolic diseases, including heart disease, type 2 diabetes, cancer and dementia. Some studies show that even three months of lifestyle change and stress reduction may have an effect on people in middle age and on genes that are involved in the ageing process. In other words stress reduction may also slow down biological ageing.

In the 21-day plan I will share Sherezade Ruano's simple guidance for how to reduce stress, which has proven to be extremely powerful in managing patients with heart disease. Unfortunately, stress management is not yet a part of routine cardiac rehabilitation in the NHS and this must change. The science is strong that managing stress through regular mindfulness practice combined with a healthy diet and exercise appears to be a crucial component for good metabolic health and longevity.

What about sleep?

Just as stress makes us feel unwell, poor sleep is something we can all relate to. There's extensive research pointing to poor sleep being a risk factor for many diseases and conditions that include high blood pressure, type 2 diabetes, heart disease, obesity and depression. We've all experienced how good and energised we feel after a good night's sleep and how just one bad night can put us at the opposite end of the spectrum.

After one night of restricted or broken sleep we may perform poorly all round and have a greater propensity to make poor food choices throughout the day.

Research suggests that we should be averaging at least seven hours' sleep per night. The 21-day plan will give you tips for exactly what you can do to maximise the chances of it. So let's get started!

CHAPTER 10

The 21-Day Immunity Plan

Why 21 days?

There are three main reasons for writing a plan for 21 days. The first is that for most people it takes three weeks to break any habit, or for many what is a form of addiction to sugar and ultra-processed food. I follow my own advice and when I started my own plan several years ago I was amazed at how my cravings for sugary foods and refined high-glycaemic index carbohydrates disappeared. After that it just seemed so much easier to keep going on a healthy path, especially as I felt better. And I consistently see this replicated in the patients I prescribe this plan to as well. This is the most important first step to set you on a path that you can then go on to build upon.

The second reason is that most people with adverse metabolic health will start to see marked improvements to their health and/ or shape albeit to different degrees within three weeks, without having to count calories.

The third reason is an important one, not just for patients but for doctors too. It is the need to change the narrative around the impact of lifestyle changes and show that their effect on health can be rapid and substantial. We should use this to motivate ourselves to continue to reap the benefits of improved health for life.

So the 21-day immunity plan is one that involves nutritious food, helps regulate and reduce inflammation, combat insulin resistance and overall improves metabolic health. It should be enjoyable and be in keeping with all cultures and personal preferences. It will help you to:

- lose excess body fat in a sustainable and enjoyable way, which will improve metabolic health irrespective of weight loss.
- support normal immune function and make you more resilient to fight infection through food, nutrition and lifestyle measures.
- reduce the risk of developing type 2 diabetes; help control blood glucose and the need for medications for those with the condition; and potentially reverse or send it into remission.
- reduce high medication loads and prevent and manage heart disease.
- get you on the road to significantly reducing your risk of developing dementia and cancer.

That said, although many people see some initial major improvements in their metabolic health, these may not be enough either to get their type 2 diabetes into remission or get to the level of weight they wish to achieve. In this instance I suggest seeking extra help from a registered dietitian, nutritionist or nutritional therapist. You may need to look at your overall calorie intake, for example, tailored to your dietary preferences. The same goes for all the other goals you're trying to achieve – you may need more specialist input from a personal trainer, psychologist or someone with expertise in stress reduction. Don't blame yourself if you're not seeing the results you want. Get extra help.

Over the course of the three weeks, you will follow an eating plan, you will be required to move your body daily, carry out breathing exercises, monitor and improve your sleep habits and be seeking to reduce your stress and improve your mental well-being by making a concerted effort to nurture and celebrate time with friends and family.

Please note that if you suffer from type 2 diabetes, high blood pressure or heart disease and more specifically are taking medications, you must consult your doctor before starting the 21-day plan, as medication will likely need adjusting/reducing and even potentially being stopped altogether.

EAT

Enjoy
- Three meals per day maximum, and eating only until you feel full. Take your time eating, eat with others if you can and enjoy your food.
- At least 2–4 tablespoons of extra virgin olive oil (EVOO) daily.
- One small handful of tree nuts (walnuts/almonds/hazelnuts/ macadamias) daily.
- At least 5–7 portions of a variety of fibrous vegetables and low-sugar fruits a day (see box below). I suggest a maximum of two pieces of low-sugar fruit and/or one medium-sugar fruit, and at least five portions of vegetables a day. Fibrous

foods tend to make you feel full for longer, reduce a rapid rise in blood glucose and insulin and are good for gut bacteria (the microbiome).
- Vegetables in at least two meals daily.
- Oily fish (such as salmon, mackerel, tuna, herring and sardines) at least three times a week.

What fruit and veg should I be eating?

Fibrous vegetables include cauliflower, broccoli, asparagus, aubergine, spinach, onions, peppers, Brussels sprouts, mushrooms, cucumber, celery, tomatoes and courgettes (tomatoes are technically a fruit, although most people think they're a vegetable). You can also eat these freely.

Low-sugar fruits include all berries, such as blueberries, raspberries and strawberries, avocados, lemons and apricots (one portion is 80g in weight; eat a maximum of two portions per day).

Medium-sugar fruits are apples, pears, oranges, peaches (eat a maximum of one per day).

Avoid
- All added sugars, fruit juice, honey and syrups. For the 21 days I advise that you go completely cold turkey on added sugar and sucrose (which is made up of 50% glucose and 50% fructose). It's the fructose component which has been

shown in scientific studies to increase liver fat and insulin resistance when consumed in excess. This is bascially food items containing sugar that lack fibre. Whole fruit in general is not a problem but for metabolic health be mindful of not consuming too many of the high-sugar fruits, especially if you're not undertaking regular vigorous activity. High sugar fruits include bananas, grapes, pineapple, mangoes and cherries.

- The World Health Organization set an ideal maximum limit of no more than 6 teaspoons of added sugar, fruit juice, syrups and honey for the average adult per day. The US Department of Agriculture recommends no more than 3 teaspoons for the average 4–8-year-old child. To put this into perspective one regular-sized chocolate bar, a glass of fruit juice or a can of cola contains almost three times that amount!

- Avoid all low-quality carbohydrates and starchy foods that lack fibre (see page 76). This includes all packaged carbo-hydrates, pastries, cakes, biscuits, muesli bars, packaged noodles, pasta, couscous and rice.

- I also recommend avoiding all grains for the 21 days of the plan because these foods, particularly rice, wheat, oats and all breads, tend to be high in starch that still significantly raise blood glucose for those who are insulin resistant. One of the most nutritious alternatives that doesn't tend to spike blood glucose is quinoa. For the 21 days, substitute rice for cauli-flower rice (available in most supermarkets) and pasta for courgetti or celeriac.

- Avoid all ultra-processed foods. If it comes in a packet and has five or more ingredients, especially if containing additives and preservatives, don't eat it.

FAST

Intermittent fasting or time-restricted eating has become a big topic in recent years, as a means of improving health and longevity. The science is rooted in experiments on rodents, which reveal that restriction of calories over their lifetime resulted in a longer lifespan.

At a very basic level intermittent fasting allows the body to use up stored energy, by burning up excess body fat. During periods of prolonged fasting, such as 16 or even 24 hours, the body switches from using glucose as its primary source of fuel to using fat in the form of ketones.

Again although intermittent fasting may help you lose weight, a number of studies have shown that many of the benefits of intermittent fasting are independent of weight loss. They include improvements in lowering insulin, controlling blood glucose levels, lowering blood pressure, aiding abdominal fat loss and enhancing exercise endurance. In other words fasting improves metabolic health.

As the data on lifespan extension of intermittent fasting is limited to animal studies, it's not definitive as to whether this applies to humans – but the case is very compelling.

For the purposes of the 21-day plan, whether you choose to fast or not is up to you and depends on where you're starting from in terms of overhauling your diet. If you find the changes above a bit daunting then I suggest you wait for a few weeks before trying it. If and when you feel confident that you can introduce it into your daily routine, then I would suggest you do so over a few weeks by gradually reducing the time window in which you eat from 12 hours to 8 hours. What you're ultimately aiming for is to fast for

16 hours per day, i.e. for your eating window to be between 10am and 6pm; 11am and 7pm or 12pm to 8pm. During that 8-hour window I suggest you eat according to your hunger levels, still sticking with the plan to avoid ultra-processed foods and refined carbohydrates. If you feel you need to eat three meals in that short time frame, that's fine, but many people get by just with two and they include some healthy snacks in between.

Be aware that when you make this switch you may experience hunger, irritability and impaired ability to concentrate during the fasting period. These side effects usually disappear within a month, so don't give up too early! During the fasting you can still have as many non-caloric drinks as you like, such as water, black coffee, green tea or herbal teas. If you're particularly stressed, however, I suggest you keep caffeine to a minimum and choose decaffeinated options.

MOVE

Our bodies are designed to move, and movement plays an integral role in sustaining our health and vitality. Not moving enough affects our muscles, resulting in reduced strength, size and function. As we discussed in the chapter about exercise (see page 63), we also know that prolonged sitting and being more sedentary in general increases the risk of heart disease, high blood pressure and type 2 diabetes. The key to keeping your body in shape is to add more movement into your daily routine.

Regular cardiovascular exercise has the strongest evidence base when it comes to reducing the risk of many diseases. It has even been shown to significantly reduce insulin resistance within three months for those who start off with a sedentary lifestyle, even without weight loss.

Throughout the three weeks of this plan, I want you to go for a brisk walk for at least 30 minutes on 5 days each week. Subjectively this is where you feel a bit out of breath to the point you're able to have a conversation but you'll find it difficult to sing. If you want to be very precise then measuring your heart rate provides a more objective measure of activity intensity. Are you doing too little or are you doing too much? You want to aim to get your heart rate within a range of 50–70% of your maximum, which is related to your age. The reason for this heart rate range is based on numerous studies which reveal beneficial physiological changes in the body start to occur once you exercise at this level, including reduced insulin resistance.

To calculate this range, you deduct your age from 220. For example, if you're aged 40 then the figure would be 180. You will need to aim to get your heart rate working at between 50–70% of that number, which in this instance is 90–126 beats per minute. For those of South Asian origin this should be a bare minimum (because of a genetic tendency towards reduced cardiorespiratory fitness) and if you have metabolic syndrome or a family history of it then you will need to add an extra 10–15 minutes to the length of time you walk, so that means 40–45 minutes 5 times per week.

If you're starting to exercise like this for the first time then perhaps start in bouts of 10 minutes per day and build up gradually over a few weeks. Listen to your body; if you start to feel exhausted, your body is telling you that you're overdoing it.

You're aiming to move as much as you can. Do not sit for more than 45 minutes at a time – take 2-minute movement breaks. I suggest getting up and doing ten squats. Take the stairs wherever possible and most importantly move in ways that you enjoy, whether it be dancing, cycling or even having sex.

BREATHE

As we now know, psychological stress is a significant contributing risk factor in up to 90% of all chronic diseases but the human body and mind can quickly achieve balance and freedom from stress by using a holistic approach. For the plan, I am going to use a tool that is freely available to all of us: our breath. Focusing on one's breathing is one of the easiest and best ways to activate the part of the nervous system that is involved in reducing stress – the parasympathetic nervous system. Even within just a few seconds of deliberately slowing one's breath, our heart rate will also slow, which is a powerful demonstration of how much the mind affects the body. Specific breathing techniques, combined with body awareness and mindfulness, can ease our mind into a state that promotes healing and recharging, so the breathing exercise below is one that I suggest you do every day throughout the 21-day plan. It was recommended to me by cardiac specialist nurse and stress reduction expert Sherezade Ruano.

Choose a comfortable position that allows you to let go of any tension – allow your body to choose the position intuitively – if you find it easier to lie down, which is what I do, then that's fine too.

Start by paying attention to where your breath is located; notice if you are breathing with your belly or using the upper chest. When you exhale, gently soften the shoulders and allow them to let go of the tension. Free up the neck by gently creating micro-movements from right to left. When you feel ready, softly close your eyes and let your body sink into a deep state of stillness. Notice how your skin starts to let go of the tension too. Gently direct your awareness towards the lower portion of your ribcage and notice the gentle sideways movement as you inhale and exhale. Focus on the softness of your breath and avoid creating resistance at the end of the inhalation. This exercise is all about letting go, so there is no need for thoughts about creating the perfect practice. There is no ideal practice but the enjoyment of noticing how our nervous system, mind and outer world slow down. Notice the subtle sensations that occur when you become an observer of your breath, with no judgments and no expectations. You are now practising mindfulness of the breath by simply allowing your mind to focus on a certain area on your body.

If you prefer something more directed and would prefer to use specific breathing techniques to focus your mind, as I do, you can either just breathe in slowly counting for five seconds in your head and then breathe out. Another technique which I find very helpful is to breathe in for four seconds through your nose, hold it for seven and then exhale for eight seconds. Counting this in your head also helps focus the mind away from any distractions.

I suggest you start by doing a breathing exercise such as these for 10 minutes every day and slowly building up to 20 and even 30 minutes. You can do this any time of day. I personally do it first thing in the morning.

SOCIALISE

Make an effort to increase time spent with friends and family each week. It's not just good for our mental health but helps mitigate stress too. Research reveals that having meaningful relationships is the biggest predictor of happiness and is also linked to health and longevity.

SLEEP

You want to be aiming to achieve a minimum of 7 hours each night. Research reveals that once you drop below this level then insulin resistance starts to increase. The overall lifestyle changes that incorporate a good diet, regular moderate exercise and mindfulness meditation, all of which are part of this plan, will also lead to a longer and more productive sleep.

Stress and sleep are very closely linked. The major cause of poor sleep is stress (see page 71), so you need to find ways of mitigating your own stresses through activities such as mindfulness meditation and regular moderate exercise. Try to switch off from social media and computer screens at least two hours before bed – this helps to reduce the type of brain activity that keeps you overstimulated and awake. Avoid caffeine after lunchtime, especially if your sleep is already poor, as the stimulant effect of caffeine can continue for many hours after your last cup.

Addressing some popular myths about this kind of plan

Can I eat red meat?

The World Cancer Research Fund recommends a maximum weekly limit of 500g per week of red meat and if possible, less of the processed forms, such as bacon. Although there is no strong link to heart disease there are concerns that consuming quantities above this level this could increase the risk of colon cancer. I advise sticking within these limits so that red meat does not replace the foods that form the base of the 21-day plan and all their positive health benefits. From a nutritional point of view red meat is still an excellent source of protein, iron and vitamin B12, so you can enjoy a juicy 200g steak or a lamb curry during the week and perhaps a weekend fry-up with a couple of rashers of bacon or sausages.

Is this a high-saturated-fat diet?

The saturated fats you are being encouraged to stop eating are those that are in ultra-processed foods, such as pies, pastries, cakes and biscuits. Foods that are high in saturated fat also include butter, full-fat dairy, cheese and red meat; however, these foods are nutritious and can be included as part of a healthy diet. As long as you get the base of the diet right, by eating plenty of fibrous vegetables, extra virgin olive oil, nuts, seeds and oily fish, there is no reason to place extra restrictions on them, especially as you're eating until full and not over-eating. It's very unlikely that this diet will take you into any concerning levels of saturated fat intake. Furthermore, the most up-to-date evidence reveals that as part of a whole-foods diet there is no strong link between the consumption of such foods and heart disease.

Will this diet have an adverse effect on my cholesterol?

No. It will almost certainly improve your cholesterol profile, depending where you're starting from. The kind of diet I'm recommending will, for the overwhelming majority of people, reduce triglycerides and raise HDL-C because this ratio strongly correlates with insulin resistance which is what we're aiming to improve.

Is there too little fibre in this diet?

On the contrary it will give you more than enough fibre because the base of the diet is high-quality carbohydrates coming from fibrous vegetables. Published research done by eminent dietitian Caryn Zinn looked at the nutrient profile and fibre content of two typical diet plans similar to the one that you'll end up adopting in the 21-day immunity plan. The fibre content was well above the recommended daily intake of 30g per day, which most people are not achieving.

Can I eat beans and other pulses?

Beans, chickpeas and lentils are very much allowed as they're nutrient-dense and full of protein and fibre.

What about salt?

Salt consumption is an ongoing area of controversy. For years we've been told to keep salt consumption to a minimum because of its link to raising high blood pressure. Cardiovascular research scientist James Di-Nicolantonio has researched this area extensively and concluded that insulin resistance is a much more important predictor than salt, and once this is corrected then salt doesn't have much effect, if any, on blood pressure.

Although, as I've seen with a small minority of my own patients, even having corrected insulin resistance and reversed many markers of metabolic syndrome, blood pressure can still remain on the high side and once salt is reduced it drops considerably. So providing you've cut out the ultra-processed food and fast food (which is where many of us get most of the salt in our diet) and low-quality carbs, you can eat salt to taste. If, however, you see your blood pressure creeping up or it's not coming down then I suggest you significantly reduce salt intake for a month and see if it makes any difference.

Can I snack between meals?

If you're following the plan and eating until fullness, but not over-eating, you shouldn't feel the need to snack. If you do then opt for a healthy nutritious snack, such as a handful of nuts or a small piece of cheese.

Can I consume alcohol?

As a nation we're consuming way too much. Alcohol in excess has a similar metabolic effect on the body as sugar. It's good to have a few days completely off alcohol per week but if you do like a tipple, then you should stick to the current recommended limit of 14 units a week and drink like they do in the Mediterranean – no more than a glass of red wine with your evening meal, which at that dose may even provide a benefit in protecting your heart.

If I'm vegetarian or vegan can I follow the 21-day plan?

Yes, although if you're vegan don't forget you'll most likely need a vitamin B12 supplement (see page 58).

CHAPTER 11

What Do I Do After 21 Days?

If it's going well and you're starting to see results, just carry on. In terms of type 2 diabetes remission the maximum effect for most is seen in up to 70 days of following a dietary plan such as this one.

In terms of metabolic health measurements, you can measure them immediately after 21 days with your doctor or health practitioner and then have a conversation with them on when is the next feasible time to re-check all five metabolic health markers (see page 12). This can be every three months, six months or even a year. Also know your vitamin D status by having it checked by your doctor as deficiency is so prevalent, especially in those from ethnic minority backgrounds, and is linked to a number of adverse health outcomes.

Educate your friends and family and consider discussing your goals with your doctor. Explain what you're doing and why. If you feel you've been helped then you may feel inspired to help others. One of my patients told me that two of his firefighter colleagues adopted such a plan and saw quite dramatic improvements in their health. One lost six stone within three months and another reversed his type 2 diabetes and lowered his blood pressure enough to resume work.

I started and have followed such a plan religiously since 2015. I lost a stone around my waist and besides needing at times to implement extra stress reduction measures, my metabolic health has been excellent. Does that mean that I don't indulge in the occasional treat? Absolutely not. Although I don't crave ultra-processed food or sugar any more, I will still occasionally indulge in a pizza with a sourdough base, or a chicken biryani takeaway at the weekend. In essence, low-quality carbohydrates now make up less than 10% of my total calorie consumption. On a population level, recent data from the US reveals low-quality carbs make up 42% of the diet – that's clearly way too much.

If this is to become a lifestyle that you follow easily and maintain, then I advise sticking to the 80/20 rule. Follow the plan at least 80% of the time and *if* you want a different kind of treat, such as a sweet desert, a takeaway or a different kind of carbohydrate, such as whole grains, rice or bread, you can indulge in them 20% of the time without feeling guilty if you do. After all, food is to be enjoyed and be a pleasure – and it can be equally enjoyable in a healthy way. But steer clear of ultra-processed foods completely.

Last but not least, why many people find it difficult to sustain a healthy lifestyle and the reason we're in this battle for our health isn't just because of misplaced dietary advice and lack of nutrition knowledge among most doctors but also very much because of the most important driver of our eating behaviours: the food environment. On a population level, sorting this out will help all of us to sustain healthier choices – and that's where the role of government and policy makers comes in.

CHAPTER 12

Better Health For All

'For medicine to achieve its greatest task it must enter the political and social life.'

—*Rudolf Virchow, German physician (1821–1902)*

No one chooses to have poor metabolic health, making them vulnerable to infection or chronic disease. As revealed by an OECD international poll, the public consider their health to be what matters most to them in life.

So how can this be equated with the fact that 80% of adults in the UK have excess body fat or 7 out of 8 American adults have poor metabolic health? As pointed out in the *New England Journal of Medicine*, 'food choices are often automatic and made without full conscious awareness.' Despite wishing to lose weight, for example, we're still tempted to buy the chocolate bar at the checkout till.

The food industry has used cleverly thought-out marketing to exploit such impulses, which are determined by people's emotional urges. They have saturated our environment with cheap, addictive ultra-processed food, making such items available to anyone, anywhere, at any time so that exercising personal responsibility becomes impossible. (Often children are deliberately targeted with their marketing and messaging and parents find it difficult to refuse the emotional demands.) To practise refusal one needs knowledge, choice, access and affordability. But as you've learned, education around the impact of food on health is poorly implemented and the food industry, who are driven by sales as opposed to looking after your health, have even influenced international dietary guidelines.

In the UK, the current NHS Eatwell Guide, which claims to be based on the best independent advice on what constitutes a healthy diet, not only has a number of ultra-processed foods on the example plate itself, but also has crisps, chocolates and cakes in the guide with vague advice to 'eat less often and in small amounts'.

The food industry spends hundreds of millions of dollars globally on marketing cheap, nutritionally poor ultra-processed food and drink. For example, in the UK in 2017, the food industry spent £143 million on advertising crisps, confectionery and sugary drinks, more than 27 times the government expenditure on healthy eating campaigns. Products are sold under the guise of being better for us, like 'fat free' or cereals 'proven to lower cholesterol' but are in fact ultra-processed and also loaded with staggering amounts of sugar. These are often foods that cause your blood glucose to rise with each serving, don't nourish you, make you feel hungry again and continue the cycle, gradually worsening your metabolic health and setting you up for chronic disease.

Education alone for individuals has a limited impact when the food environment is working so hard against you. As the Centres of Disease Control and Prevention's health impact pyramid created by Dr Tom Frieden reveals, making the default choice the healthy choice has a far greater impact on population health than individual counselling or education.

And for many of the most vulnerable members of society, even if empowered with the right information, healthy food is unaffordable and understandably not a priority when they struggle with the psychological stress of job insecurity, low wages and poor housing, which in themselves drive poor diet, being sedentary, depression and dependence on alcohol, so fuelling metabolic disease, misery and premature death. And when it comes to maldistribution of resources in our healthcare system, the current Secretary of State for Health and Social Care, Matt Hancock, has said, 'Each year we are spending £97 billion of public money on treating disease and only £8 billion in preventing it – that's an imbalance in urgent need of correction.' And such statements do reflect the evidence. In the US, for example, people living in areas of high Medicare spend have neither improved patient satisfaction nor better health outcomes. In fact, death rates are slightly worse. The evidence is clear: the power of modern medicine is dwarfed by the power of prevention and the wider determinants of health, such as dietary choices and lifestyle.

Identifying the problem and understanding the science is half the battle but what are the solutions?

For decades after the first links between smoking and lung cancer were made, the smoking lobby were able to avoid just regulation by planting doubt that cigarettes were harmful, confusing the public, buying the loyalty of scientists and political allies and even asserting downright denial.

Eventually, when this was all exposed, regulations were introduced and tobacco consumption massively reduced across the population. In fact, the biggest factor behind the decline in cardiovascular mortality in the last three decades was witnessed after policy changes that addressed the affordability, availability and the *acceptability* of smoking. Raising the price of cigarettes had the greatest effect on the reduction in smoking, for example – and within one year of the public smoking ban being implemented in Scotland there was a 17% reduction in hospital admissions for heart attack.

From what we know about poor diet and ultra-processed food I have no doubt that government policies based on the above principles will start to have a strong and rapid impact within an even shorter timeframe than cigarettes. We know dietary changes alone can reverse metabolic syndrome in 21 days. And in the longer term, a prediction study in the US suggests that a 30 per cent subsidy on fruit and vegetables would prevent almost 2 million heart attacks and strokes over a lifetime and simultaneously save about $40 billion in healthcare costs. Yet most of us are not aware of all the system failures that perpetuate the status quo and cause avoidable misery and premature deaths of millions around the globe every year.

To be armed with this information, knowing the gross injustice that is being inflicted on our patients, members of the public, especially the most vulnerable members of society, and the majority of my doctor and allied healthcare staff colleagues, and not act on it makes us part of the problem. Therefore, it is also our duty and responsibility to act. It doesn't have to be this way. Below are my ten key points for government and policy makers, but as a member of the public you can be an advocate for these changes too.

1. Taxation of all ultra-processed foods and drinks needs to be enforced with the money gained going directly to subsidise whole and minimally processed foods, such as fruit and vegetables

2. All medical students and doctors need to have adequate training in nutrition and lifestyle medicine.

3. Every doctor should be measuring the metabolic health of their patients and making lifestyle prescriptions specifically linked to diet, physical activity and stress reduction to improve those health markers as their first-line intervention *before* the use of medication.

4. Compulsory nutrition education and cooking skills introduced into all school curriculums.

5. All hospital chief executives need to be made accountable for allowing the sale and promotion of ultra-processed food on hospital grounds, as it continues to harm the health of staff and patients and legitimises the acceptability of such food consumption to the wider public.

6. A ban on the advertising of all ultra-processed food and drink on television and online on-demand services.

7. A public education campaign is needed to help consumers understand what ultra-processed food is and the harm it causes.

8. A complete ban and disassociation of ultra-processed food and drink sponsorship of sports teams and sporting events.

9. Local authorities should encourage active travel and protect and increase green spaces in urban areas to make the healthy option the easy option.

10. Medical staff, including doctors, nurses and dietitians, should themselves be assessed on their metabolic health and

encouraged and helped to improve it, not just to set an example to patients but to optimise their own health and performance.

The above recommendations are based on evidence but also on fairness and justice for the sake of everyone's health. Armed with the knowledge in this book, if we ALL collectively advocate for these changes we'll get far closer to creating an environment where everyone, regardless of class, colour or creed, has a much better and brighter chance of living a healthy and happy life. Time for action on metabolic health and investment in well-being is long overdue. If we don't act, there may be even more misery and devastation when the next pandemic comes around.

One thing the COVID-19 crisis has taught us is that we're all interconnected and rely on each other to be able to live our lives to the fullest. In his book *A Monk's Guide to Happiness*, Gelong Thubten explains this in simple terms: 'All of the objects we use, such as our food and clothing, have been made for us by others. Because of interdependence everyone has been part of the creation of those things.'

Let's start by making it our collective responsibility to ensure that everyone has easy access to nutritious, healthy food.

References

Chapter 1

https://jamanetwork.com/journals/jama/fullarticle/2768391, accessed 20 July 2020

Chapter 2

https://www.cdc.gov/mmwr/preview/mmwrhtml/00056796.htm, accessed 20 July 2020

Chapter 3

https://www.americashealthrankings.org/learn/reports/2015-annual -report/comparison-nations-2, accessed 20 July 2020

https://www.liebertpub.com/doi/10.1089/met.2018.0105, accessed 20 July 2020

https://pubmed.ncbi.nlm.nih.gov/25355584/, accessed 20 July 2020 https://www.bmj.com/too-much-medicine, accessed 20 July 2020

https://dmsjournal.biomedcentral.com/articles/10.1186/1758-5996-6-12, accessed 20 July 2020

https://www.cochrane.org/CD006742/HTN_benefits-of-antihypertensive-drugs-for-mild-hypertension-are-unclear, accessed 20 July 2020

Chapter 4

https://academic.oup.com/advances/article/7/1/66/4524061, accessed 20 July 2020

https://www.europeanscientist.com/en/article-of-the-week/covid-19-and-the-elephant-in-the-room/, accessed 20 July 2020

https://www.ncbi.nlm.nih.gov/pmc/articles/PMC3354930/, accessed 20 July 2020

https://www.ncbi.nlm.nih.gov/pmc/articles/PMC5291468/, accessed 20 July 2020

https://www.ageuk.org.uk/globalassets/age-uk/documents/reports-and-publications/reports-and-briefings/health--wellbeing/rb_april11_evidence_review_healthy_ageing.pdf, accessed 20 July 2020

Chapter 5

https://www.thelancet.com/journals/lancet/article/PIIS0140-6736(19)30041-8/fulltext

https://www.mdpi.com/2072-6643/12/7/1955, accessed 20 July 2020

https://www.cell.com/cell-metabolism/pdf/S1550-4131(19)30248
-7.pdfhttps://academic.oup.com/ajcn/article/94/2/479/4597872,
accessed 20 July 2020

https://www.bmj.com/content/361/bmj.k2340, accessed 20 July 2020

Chapter 6

https://www.ncbi.nlm.nih.gov/pmc/articles/PMC6471908/, accessed
20 July 2020

https://openheart.bmj.com/content/2/1/e000273, accessed 20 July
2020

https://www.ncbi.nlm.nih.gov/pmc/articles/PMC3230082/, accessed
20 July 2020

https://insight.jci.org/articles/view/128308, accessed 20 July 2020

https://journals.physiology.org/doi/pdf/10.1152/japplphys-
iol.01292.2005, accessed 20 July 2020

Chapter 7

https://nutrition.bmj.com/content/early/2020/06/17/bmjnph-2020
-000100, accessed 20 July 2020

https://nutrition.bmj.com/content/early/2020/05/20/bmjnph-2020
-000085, accessed 20 July 2020

Chapter 8

https://pubmed.ncbi.nlm.nih.gov/31193280/, accessed 20 July 2020

https://www.aomrc.org.uk/reports-guidance/exercise-the-miracle
-cure-0215/, accessed 20 July 2020

https://bjsm.bmj.com/content/49/15/967, accessed 20 July 2020

https://www.bbc.co.uk/news/health-32417699, accessed 20 July 2020

Chapter 9

https://www.ncbi.nlm.nih.gov/pmc/articles/PMC5476783/, accessed
20 July 2020

Chapter 11

https://bmjopen.bmj.com/content/8/2/e018846.info, accessed 20
July 2020

https://www.nejm.org/doi/full/10.1056/NEJMra1905136, accessed 20
July 2020

https://jamanetwork.com/journals/jama/fullarticle/2751719,
accessed 20 July 2020

Chapter 12

https://jamanetwork.com/journals/jama/fullarticle/2767353,
accessed 20 July 2020

Acknowledgements

I'm very grateful for the constructive comments given to me in the book from Professor Robert Lustig, Dr Campbell Murdoch, Dr Caryn Zinn, Dr Duane Mellor and Kim Pearson.

'This game-changing book is a must-read for anyone wishing to understand the link between metabolic health and immunity.'

Dr Ravi Kumar Kamepalli, Board-Certified in Infectious Diseases, Wound Care and Obesity Medicine, Augusta, USA

'Dr Aseem Malhotra has clearly and concisely communicated the science and rationale underlying this preventable modern epidemic and has given us an easy to follow prescription, free from medication, that can reverse many of the world's ills. It's a two-hour read that might just save your life.'

Dr James Muecke AM, 2020 Australian of the Year

'Dr Aseem Malhotra spells it all out right here in front of you, with a perfect combination of smart, simple strategies for prevention or management of lifestyle conditions and keeping the immune system in best shape.'

Dr Caryn Zinn, Senior Lecturer, Dietitian, AUT University, Head of Research – School of Support and Recreation, Auckland, New Zealand

'This groundbreaking book empowers the reader with knowledge of the practical steps we can all take to improve our health status and protect ourselves against diseases of all kinds.'

Kim Pearson, Harley Street nutritionist